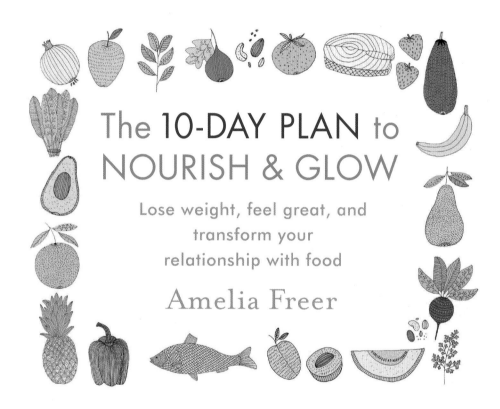

The 10-DAY PLAN to NOURISH & GLOW

Lose weight, feel great, and
transform your
relationship with food

Amelia Freer

appetite
by RANDOM HOUSE

CONTENTS

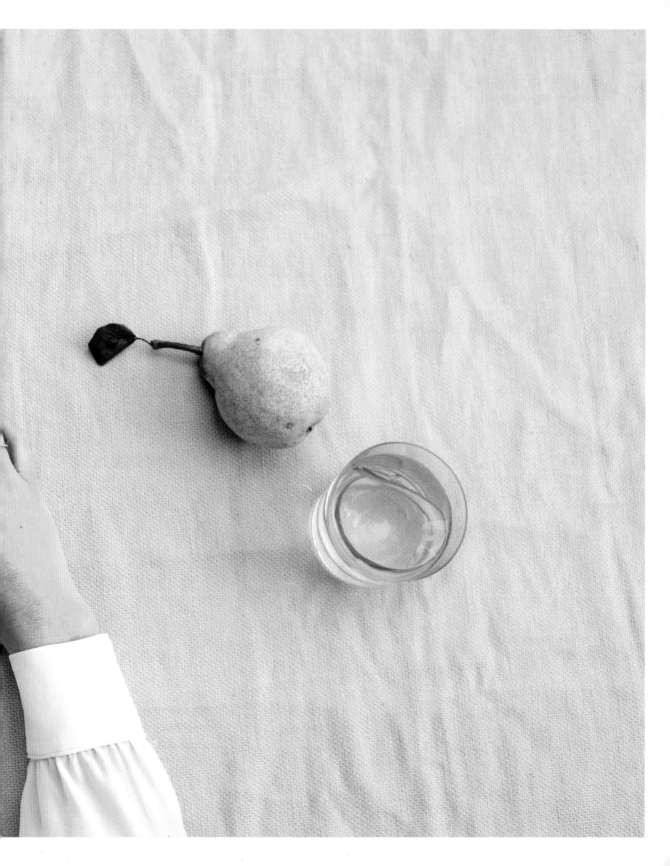

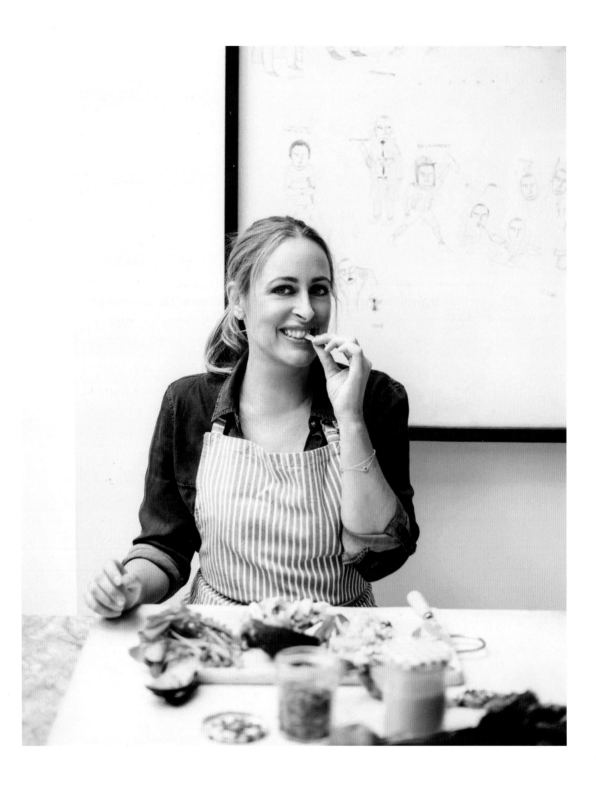

*"For what it's worth: it's never too late
to be whoever you want to be."*
—Adapted from F. Scott Fitzgerald,
The Curious Case of Benjamin Button

I have been deeply humbled by the feedback I have received from both *Eat. Nourish. Glow.* and *Cook. Nourish. Glow.* To hear that so many people have been able to move toward a healthier and more satisfying relationship with food is exactly what I set out to achieve. The community that has also been created among readers, who work tirelessly to support each other and me, is amazing to witness and I sincerely thank you all.

I would hazard a guess that by now most people (especially if you have read my previous two books!) have a fairly good idea about the general principles of healthy eating. But turning these principles into a complete meal, for a whole day, week, or even year of good food, without falling into the common pitfalls can be a little more difficult.

We also find ourselves facing a whole new set of challenges these days. The clean eating movement has swept across us as a tidal wave of marketing and media hype, bombarding us with messages about what we supposedly *must* eat and what we *must* avoid at all costs. This movement has, in some ways, been a step in the right direction—with good nutrition taking center stage and easier access to whole-food ingredients. But (and this is a big but) it has also created a lot of anxiety, fear, and confusion around food. Healthy eating has become a touchy subject.

So that is where I hope that I can help out again. Relaxed nutritional balance is how I approach my own diet and what I help my clients to achieve.

Food is not something that should be feared. Yes, it is important to eat with consciousness both for our own health and the health of the environment—but food can also be a carefree source of pleasure and joy. Identifying where our own personal balance lies on this continuum is the key to finding contentment around food.

Nourish & Glow: The 10-Day Plan is therefore not just a diet book, nor indeed just a recipe book. It is a comprehensive handbook, gently guiding you to find your own insights and building up your knowledge and skills, encouraging you to explore a way of eating healthy that is right for you.

We will explore your mind-set, habits, and how your approach to eating is influenced by family and friends, and peel away any "emotional baggage" you may be holding onto around food. You will wipe the slate clean of conflicting and confusing messages. Instead, you will learn about the concept of Positive Nutrition with a simple but effective pyramid tool. No more talk of "everything in moderation," which I hear all too often yet find to be a rather vague and unhelpful phrase for those struggling with their nutrition.

You will then have the opportunity to put this into practice by working through a carefully designed 10-day meal plan. This will enable you to find out what it really feels like to plan, shop, cook, and eat in a healthy way, while learning some simple new recipes and time-saving methods. The final chapter will help to arm you with the skills to maintain these new habits for life. These are fundamental in creating the strong foundations for a life of nourishing nutrition—yet are so often overlooked.

It is likely that there are things in these pages that will not particularly resonate with you. It is, after all, impossible to create a "one size fits all" approach when there are so many differences between us. This is one of the most misleading concepts promoted by the diet industry. Instead, I want to help you feel empowered to make your own decisions. To discard what you don't need and to try out what you do. To adapt and play with ideas. Ultimately, achieving good nutrition is a lifelong experiment of trial and error. No guru, blogger, celebrity chef, or self-styled expert can do that for you. This is your life and only you can find out what works best. But we could all do with a helping hand along the way.

This book can therefore be whatever you need it to be: a source of new recipes, some mind-set help, or a set of guidelines for meal planning among other things. Above all, I hope that it offers solutions to help move away from restrictive, negative beliefs and the cycle of being "good" or "bad" with food.

When I work with clients, this is where I start. We discuss their current lifestyle, habits, preferences, and limiting beliefs and then work together to find practical solutions. I understand that not everyone is able to work with a nutritional therapist or functional medicine practitioner (although I wish we all could). Therefore, I hope that this book can act like a surrogate nutritional therapist, bringing a bit of my practice into your home.

What a healthy diet means for you will be different from what it means for your best friend, your mother, your colleagues, or even me. And that really is the key here—because a "healthy diet" is as unique as we are.

My wonderful colleague Rozzie sums this up beautifully: "A 'healthy diet' is as unique as a fingerprint, as tailored as a Savile Row suit, and as personalized as a portrait. It's just that sometimes we need a little help to find the one that fits perfectly."

I recognize that healthy living is not always easy, and it can be made harder by the conflicting guidance we are exposed to and the individual differences between us. However, it is possible, and it is certainly important.

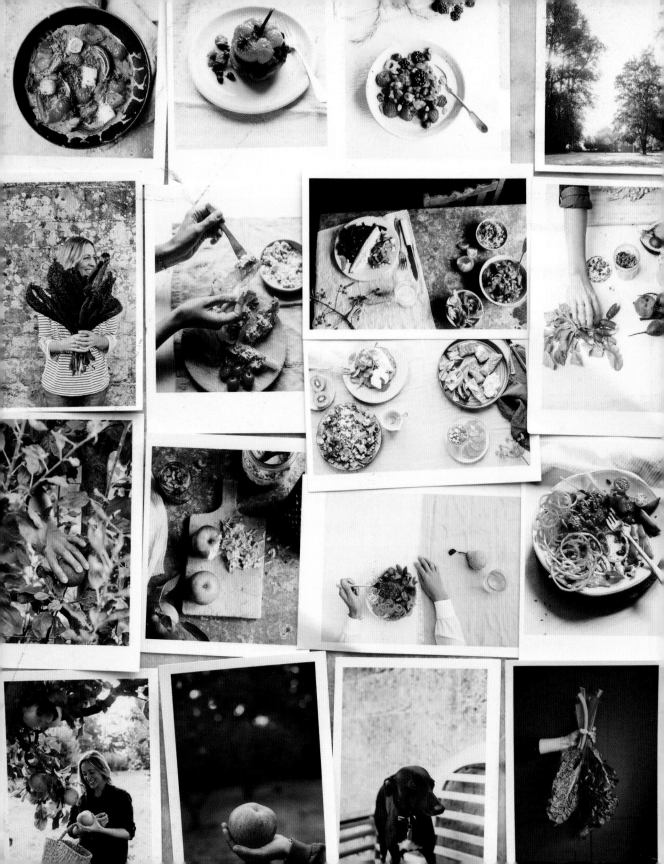

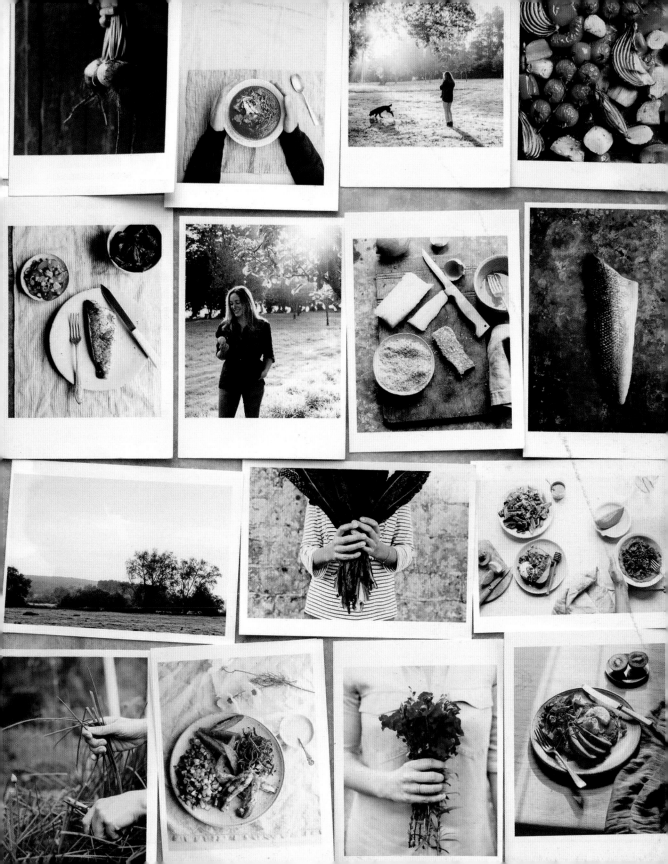

"Note to self: This journey isn't about impressing others, or fitting into a smaller dress size, or beating myself up for past mistakes. This is about honoring the extraordinary body I have been blessed with, so that I may live the life of my desires."

My aim is that this book will become a trusty companion and advisor to you, helping you to find your own way around any obstacles that may be in your path, building your confidence and enabling you to find both balance and joy from your food. The new habits that you end up making may be more subtle than you would have expected at the start—often it is the smallest changes that lead to the greatest results.

While I know that some of you will be drawn to this book because you want to lose weight, it is my sincere hope that you will be able to see its potential to change how you think and feel about food for life. I am against diets and short-term quick fixes. They never work because they don't address the core reasons why people eat food that damages them. This book is not a diet book. Yes, if you follow the 10-day plan, you may well lose weight if you have some to lose, but what will also happen—much more excitingly, in my opinion—is that you will learn how to enjoy delicious, nurturing food for life and enjoy many more health benefits far beyond what the scale says.

Give me ten days, and I hope I can help you for a lifetime.

Amelia

A healthy lifestyle is more than just a healthy diet

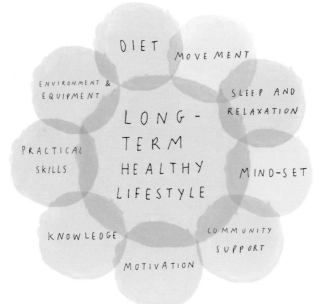

This diagram represents some of the key factors that are required to create a healthy lifestyle. And a healthy lifestyle is critical for managing weight, optimizing energy, and promoting good health.

So much advice is targeted at just one of these areas and doesn't take into consideration the balance that is necessary between them all. I know from my experience that addressing diet alone is often not enough to achieve optimal health (even though it is a great place to start). Both science and common sense have also shown us the importance of sleep, movement, community support, etc.

I have tried to address a number of different factors here—but it is beyond the scope of this book, and my expertise, to tackle them all in detail. However, I feel it's important to highlight them anyway, to give you the opportunity to reflect on your own balance and consider whether some factors may need a little more attention. Because it is only with this systematic and considered approach that we can truly set ourselves up to make long-term changes.

Chapter One:
HOW WE THINK
ABOUT WHAT WE EAT

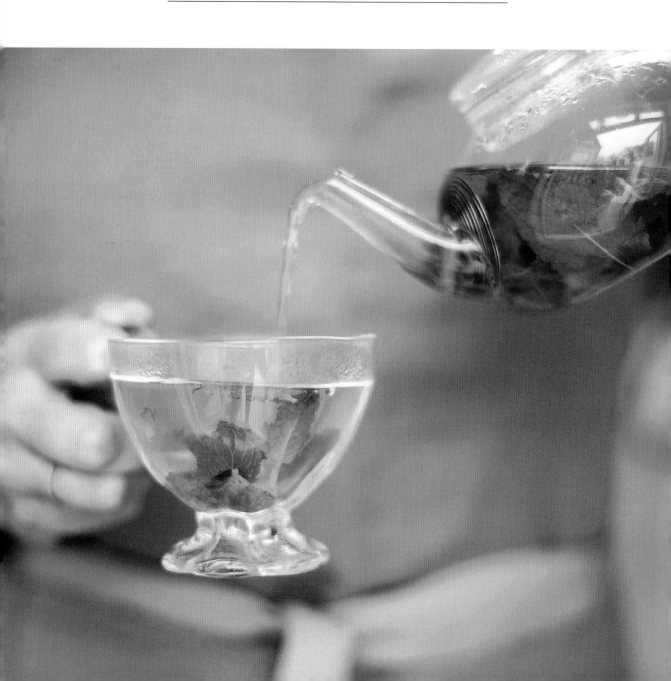

"Ability is what you're capable of doing.
Motivation determines what you do.
Attitude determines how well you do it."
—Lou Holtz

TAKING THE FIRST STEP TOWARD ANY LONG-LASTING LIFESTYLE CHANGE PROVIDES US WITH THE PERFECT OPPORTUNITY TO WORK ON OUR MIND-SET. That is not to say that we need to have worked out every last little thing that niggles at us, plays on our mind, or has troubled us in the past before starting. But a little bit of time invested early on, to help our thinking about food to be more positive and mindful, lays a strong foundation for everything else to come, and hugely increases our chance of success.

I know that lots of you might now be keen to skip straight to the nitty-gritty and leap into the 10-day meal plan rather than bothering with all the preparation stages. I am often equally eager. There is, of course, absolutely nothing stopping you from doing just that, and I am sure that you will still gain a lot from the plan. But I suggest that you pause just for a moment, and ask yourself the following questions:

1. Your past experiences

Have you ever tried to change your lifestyle in the past, only to find yourself going back to your old habits a few days, weeks, or months down the line?

2. Willpower and motivation

Do you ever find yourself "running out" of willpower or motivation?

3. Anxious and fearful when making food choices

Do you have an internal dialogue that is anxious and fearful when making food choices, or do you find yourself bewildered by all the contradictory information out there about what a healthy diet actually is?

4. "Comfort food"

Do you ever reach for "comfort food" when life is tough? Or have you ever felt you are "out of control" around food?

5. Food as expression

Is less-than-healthy food sometimes used as an expression of love in your family or to yourself? Would doing without it, or declining it, cause friction?

If you answered "yes" to any of those questions, I would urge you to slow down and try working through this book step by step. It has been designed to help tackle these challenges head-on, and by doing so, to create a more positive mind-set that is primed and ready for change. Good nutrition is just as much about our minds as it is about food.

How We Think About What We Eat

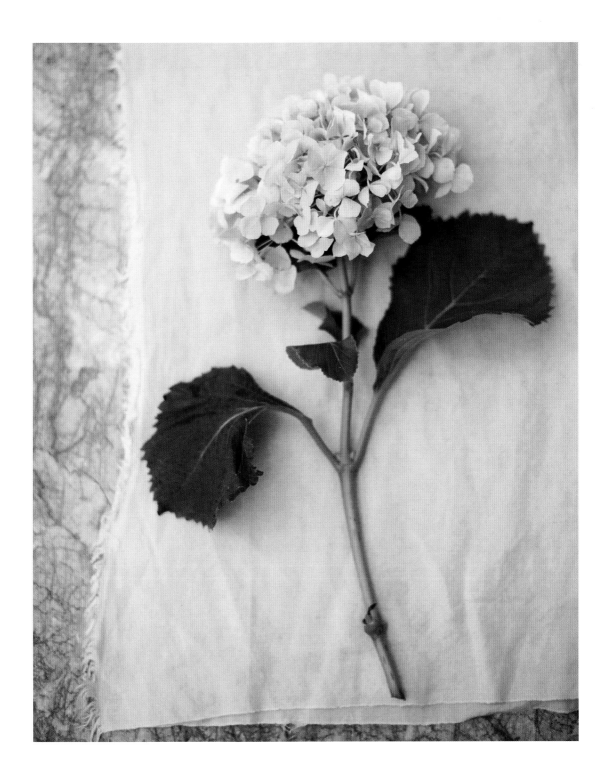

Let's start by exploring how we think about what we eat.

When it comes to finding our own balance of good nutrition, learning what works, and what doesn't, is a unique and personal journey. In my experience, it is rarely a process that can be rushed, as there is often a lot of experimentation needed along the way.

There certainly was for me anyway, and I believe in adjusting and tailoring your diet as you go along. The word "diet" means the food and drinks that we habitually consume, but its original meaning was "way of life"—and this is my main focus. Make changes, but know that nothing needs to be set in stone; notice how your body reacts; look out for changes in your energy levels, mood, sleep, and skin. I tried to be vegetarian many years ago, but it didn't suit my health, and while I would never say everyone needs to eat a certain way, I personally need some animal protein in my diet to feel really well. That said, I know that other people feel fantastic without eating animal protein, so just be aware that everybody is as individual as you are.

I also wholeheartedly believe that there is nothing wrong *at all* with taking the slow road when it comes to making changes.

Like so many people, I love food. So when I first realized I had to make changes to my diet it felt really hard and scary. For example, cutting down on my daily ten cups of tea with three sugars. I couldn't go cold turkey and had to do it slowly. I went through the same process with a number of food habits.

It is true that sometimes people with specific health conditions may need to dive in at the deep end with the radical elimination of certain foods. But I think that for most people a slow and measured approach is more likely to result in us making changes in a sustainable manner. Hares and tortoises certainly come to mind here!

Finding out what works for us is not just about the actual food that we are consuming, but also about our whole mentality. We each approach eating with a different set of emotions, memories, and cultural and family expectations behind us. In my experience, it is often these subtle influences that sneakily trip clients up—however much they consciously *want* to transform.

We are able to influence some of these factors, and some we cannot. But understanding a little more about how they might be impacting our daily habits and food choices is a fantastic start and allows us the freedom to change what we can and let go of what we can't.

Let me give you an example.

Case study: Food as Love

I was working with a woman who was significantly over what is considered to be a healthy weight. She was suffering from various health problems as a result of this, even though she was only in her thirties. A traditional approach would have been to dive right in and start giving advice about her eating habits. But in this case, that would have been learning to run before we could walk. So instead, we started at the beginning and began to explore the context of her life in much more detail. By doing so, we discovered that she used food as an expression of affection—not only to those she loved, but also to herself. This was how she had been shown love as a child, and it was an ingrained part of her family routine.

Taking away the foods associated with such strong emotions and memories without acknowledging this first would have been quite traumatic for her. It would have been setting my client up for failure before we had even started. So instead, our first step was to explore alternative ways of expressing her love and affection for herself and others, using nonfood treats. She could then cut those emotional ties to "treat" foods, leaving her free to choose alternative, healthier options.

Knowledge of our own thoughts, influences, emotions, and beliefs about food is the key to creating change, so let's explore some of these potential "tripping hazards," as I like to call them, in a little more detail.

THE HIDDEN MESSAGE:
using food as an offering of love

Eating has always been about much more than just relieving hunger. Offering and accepting gifts of food, however small, has been used as a sign of affection for those we love, as a welcome to strangers, and as an expression of religious beliefs for millennia. I love that this is true across so many continents and cultures. Food holds much more significance than just calories or taste—it also conveys infinite hidden messages.

Sharing food has even played an important role in our evolution, by increasing the closeness of our relationships and helping us to develop social bonds. If you think about it, the act of giving up your own food for someone else, particularly if you have little to spare, is an incredibly powerful way to show just how important you consider that person to be. It is a rare celebration that is not accompanied by some sort of feasting; even a business meeting offers at least coffee and cookies. Sharing food brings people, communities, and families together. We still exchange nutrition as part of making closer social connections all of the time.

But food can also be used as a more intimate expression of love. Couples often spend their free time together sharing a meal, parents bake for their children, and friends throw elaborate dinner parties for one another. If we care deeply about someone, the act of shopping, preparing, serving, or eating food can be a very powerful way of communicating our affection. Our love runs through the act of bringing food to the table and consuming it together.

As well as using food as an outward sign of love, we may also use food as our go-to gift of comfort. Just as a crying infant is soothed by the offer of milk, so we have all learned, from the earliest of ages, to associate comfort with the feeling of a full stomach. Add on to this years of bribery,

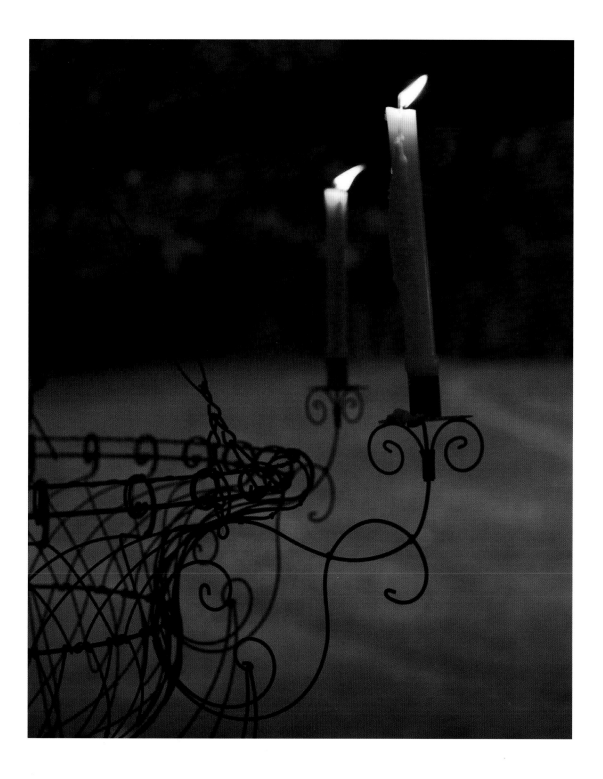

"treats," and "Oh, I deserve it!" moments, and it is no wonder that food is a security blanket for many. Wanting to extend this to others we care about is therefore no surprise.

If someone we know is upset, one of our first instincts is often to offer them a cup of tea (or something stronger!), or a slice of cake. By doing so, we are trying to make things a little better for them. Providing something to eat or drink not only acts as a distraction and comfort to the receiver, but feeling like we are able to *do* something can also make us feel better too.

I am no exception to these examples. One of my greatest pleasures in life is creating and serving food to my friends and family, and I get huge satisfaction from enjoying a meal together. And I most certainly have been known to use good food to help cheer up friends. Food is therefore very much an expression of *my* love for others. And there is absolutely nothing wrong with that.

However, I think it is still useful to bring a little mindfulness to our own experiences of food being used to convey a message. Because if we make significant, healthy changes to our food choices, this may unwittingly change the messages we are used to giving or receiving through food. We can then prepare ourselves and others for this accordingly, and the better prepared we are, the less likely we are to lose our way.

The key point about giving and receiving messages through food or drink is that although it can be a wonderfully loving and caring act, it shouldn't end up causing harm in the long term to either ourselves or others. The occasional "treat" is a joy, but when this becomes a regular habit, then perhaps we need to reevaluate things a little.

Consider, for example, a husband who always picks up a chocolate bar for his wife on the way home from work as a gift of love. This gift usually makes her happy, which makes him feel proud. If she decides one day to reject this chocolate bar, because she has started a new healthy-eating plan, how will he feel? Rejected? Perhaps guilty? Angry at the plan, and therefore not eager to support it? Maybe he will even try to sabotage the idea, albeit subconsciously.

Another example: it's finally Friday night, and you decide that after a stressful week you deserve a reward. So you head out for a few drinks, and get some takeout on the way home. If you decide to cut down on your alcohol intake and avoid takeout for a while, how will you then feel come Friday? Disappointed that you might be missing out? Sad that you haven't had your usual reward? Maybe even a little lonely? Losing motivation by the second.

Maybe you recognize yourself in these examples, or perhaps you recognize others. Either way, how can we turn what is, fundamentally, a very loving act into something that also supports the long-term health of both ourselves and those we care for?

Start off by considering whether are there any *other* ways that you could show your feelings that are not related to treat food. And how about showing affection and kindness to ourselves? Self-love through the enjoyment of healthy nourishing foods will feed a virtuous cycle of well-being for both mind and body. Turn over the page for some nonfood treat ideas that I use. I'm sure you can think of others too.

If necessary, try discussing these ideas with those closest to you ahead of time, and make clear to them that swapping your usual food treats for non-edible alternatives will not change your relationship.

Nonfood Treats

- Handwritten notes
- Tiny presents
- Flowers—even just a couple of stems picked from the garden
- Physical touch or hugs
- Words of encouragement or comfort
- A walk together
- A listening ear
- Offers of practical help
- Advice
- A long bath
- A movie or new TV show
- An evening with a good book

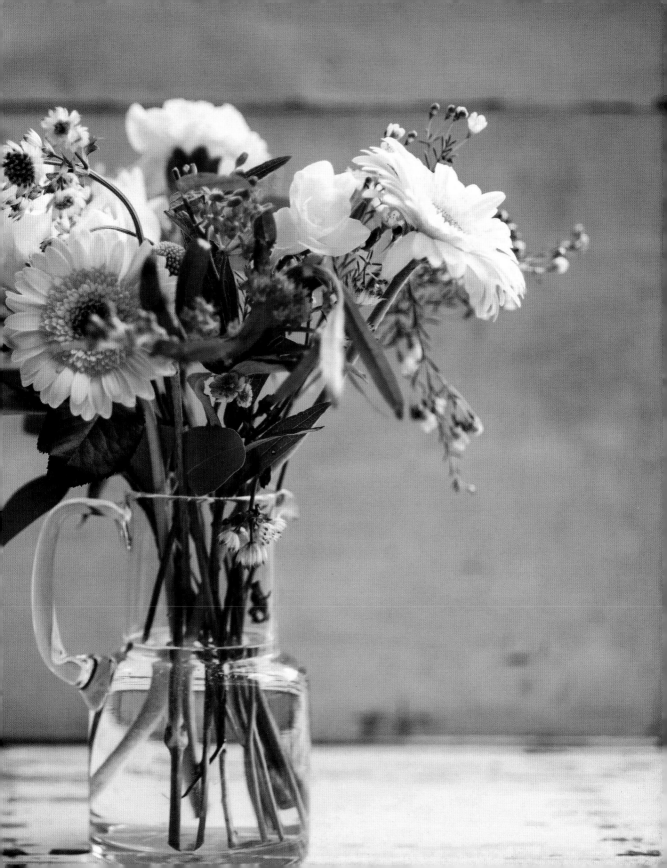

WE NEVER REALLY EAT ALONE:
the power of social influence

So much thinking about nutrition is focused on us as lone individuals. But the truth is that almost all of us are part of a larger network of people with whom we share food and dining experiences. And that wider network can have more of an impact on our eating habits than we might think.

We tend to share lots of similarities in our eating habits with the people that we are closest to. After all, we are social beings at heart and we therefore like to "fit in." We use the behavior of others to judge how we should behave, even when it comes to food. So if all of our friends party hard every weekend, we are far more likely to do the same than become a vegetarian triathlete . . . This is a silly, extreme example, but hopefully you get my point.

Although we may be unknowingly copying other people's bad habits, we can also piggy-back on their good ones. This happens not only when we are with them, but even when we are alone. It seems that the good habits of others can breed good habits in us. Do you know anyone who you feel leads a healthy lifestyle? Or do you have a friend who is keen to make healthy changes? Finding someone or a few friends you can share this experience with really helps, with both the ups and the downs. You can encourage and inspire each other to succeed.

"With life's distractions popping up from everywhere, it is easy to lose sight of this important journey."

—Jessica Semaan

If you don't have anyone specifically to go on this journey with, there are now many online resources to take inspiration from too.

Research has shown that we tend to eat more food, and faster, when we are sharing meals with people we feel very close to, whereas we may eat more slowly, and less overall, when we are dining with people we don't know so well. We can also subconsciously change how much we eat depending on the serving sizes of our dining companions. So the more others load up their plates, the more we will do the same and vice versa. Of course, there are always exceptions to any rule. From experience with my clients, I know that some people will barely eat a thing in public, however well they know the people they are eating with, but will eat much more in private. This can often be tied up with feelings of shame or embarrassment, or of being conscious of how others may view our food choices—a whole separate topic in itself.

Most of the time we may not be particularly aware of these effects, as much of it is subconscious. However, it's a good idea to bring a little mindfulness to how these social influences may be impacting our own eating habits. By all means let your hair down and enjoy yourself fully when dining in a crowd, but doing so consciously and doing so unconsciously are very different. So let's try to aim for more conscious eating.

EMOTIONAL EATING:
the constant dance between emotion and appetite

Emotions can influence our tendency to eat, and for some the effect of these on appetite and food choices can be quite striking. You probably know already if you are an "emotional eater" (but remember that this is *not* a permanent label; it comes and goes over time). We may eat for a whole range of different emotional reasons, such as boredom, anger, fear, loneliness, grief, stress, joy, or excitement.

For example, negative emotions, such as sadness, may increase our appetite and push us toward less healthy food choices, whereas joy and other positive emotions usually increase our enjoyment of food and may encourage us to eat more mindfully and healthily.

But why do negative emotions like this make us more likely to reach for junk food specifically? The "comfort food" that we turn to when we are upset is generally high in fat and sugar, and is easily eaten or prepared. Eating can firstly be a welcome distraction from our mental discomfort in the short term. But the combination of sugar and fat creates a chemical reaction in the brain that stimulates the release of "feel good" neurotransmitters. Unfortunately, this can lead to a vicious cycle of over-reliance on "comfort foods." In a way we are trying to self-medicate our negative emotions through food. In fact, sugar solutions have even been used to calm and soothe infants during medical procedures as they are so effective at comforting us.

But the problem is that this doesn't work in the long term; it just *perpetuates the vicious cycle*. The more we seek emotional comfort from food, the more it conditions us to want the same next time. It can also pile on feelings of guilt, even self-loathing—which then make us feel even worse, driving us back toward emotional eating.

When we see this in black and white, it becomes clear that this pattern of behavior is not serving our optimal health. If this is something you recognize in yourself, please rest assured that you are not alone. The cycle is really common, and really powerful. The first step to breaking it is to become aware that we are doing it. The next is to find alternative solutions to uncomfortable emotions.

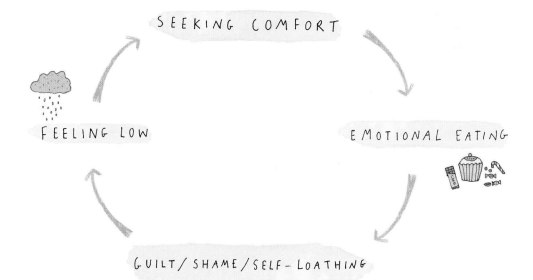

STRESSFUL FOOD: what drives overeating when the going gets tough?

"Stress" is a notoriously difficult problem to define. It affects each and every one of us differently. What overstretches one person may just be an exciting challenge for another. But in general, stress produces a feeling of vulnerability, which can have repercussions on our food choices.

People under stress may tend to overeat, undereat, or just slip into the habit of relying on ready meals or takeout food eaten in a distracted hurry. According to one report, around 30 percent of people may eat more food when stressed, while roughly 50 percent may eat less. For the remaining 20 percent, stress may have little impact on their food intake. Interestingly, it may be that this is also *regardless of weight*, with overweight or obese people no more likely than people of normal weight to resort to stress-induced eating. In other words, it can affect all of us. I know that when I am stressed, I am more likely to skip meals and stop cooking and shopping, get out of good habits and turn to lazy food options. Stress makes me lose my appreciation of food.

So what leads some people to react to an emotion by reaching for the cookie jar? The answer might be surprising, but it seems that dieting may be partly to blame, or, more specifically, limiting our energy intake in an effort to control our eating or weight. People who are dieting may be more likely to overeat when they feel stressed than people who are not on a diet. This may be particularly true for those who have been restricting what they are eating for a long time—the classic yo-yo or chronic dieters (remember, this is regardless of current weight).

What's more, the stricter your diet—the more restrained you're trying to be over your food intake—the more likely you may be to overeat in response to stress. If that alone is not an excellent reason never to crash-diet again, I am not sure what is.

Just as a side note, stress may also affect our ability to digest properly. It can slow down the absorption of glucose from the carbohydrates in our food, as well as slowing the movement of food through the digestive tract. So taking a few moments out of a busy day to sit down and enjoy our meals properly is not only a good stress-reliever in itself, but it also helps us to extract maximum nutrition from our food. Healthy food promotes calm, and vice versa.

Prioritizing some rest and relaxation may seem a big ask when you are rushed off your feet but it is crucial that you give yourself permission to do this. Only *you* know what you enjoy and what is realistic in your schedule, but I urge you to take a moment to think about this well ahead of time if you recognize that your eating habits change in response to stress, or if you are under pressure at the moment. You will thank yourself for it later. So many of my clients report that managing their stress helps them to make better food choices.

BREAKING THE CYCLE OF EMOTIONAL EATING

Here is a useful mindfulness exercise that can help us to work out whether we are seeking food because we are truly, physically hungry or because we are stressed, bored, lonely, or sad. Sometimes it can actually be quite difficult to tell the difference, particularly if we have been emotionally eating for a long time. Try this the next time that you find yourself struggling with a hunger you're not convinced is real.

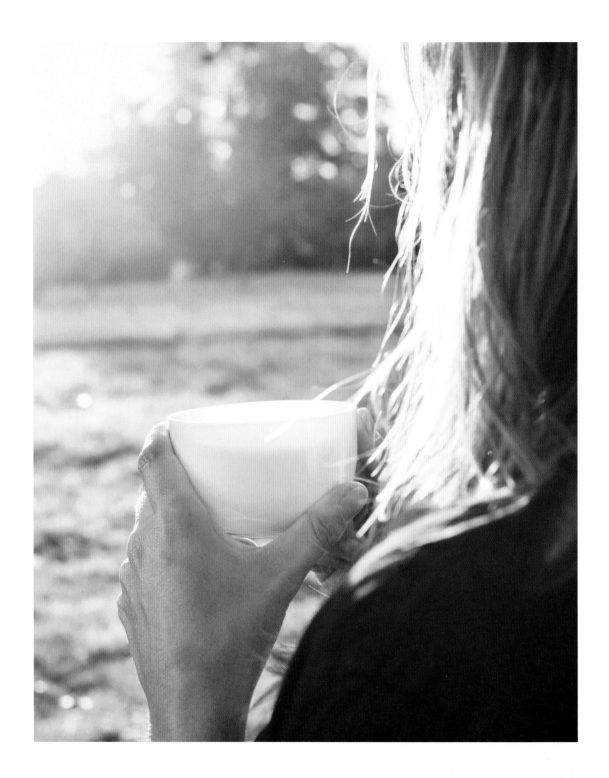

Mindful Exercise

1. *Begin by presuming that this is, in fact, a sneaky emotion in disguise and not your body saying it is hungry (assuming that you have eaten sensibly at your previous meals).*

2. *Ask yourself where exactly in your body you are feeling your hunger. Are you feeling it truly in your stomach—is it growling and rumbling? Would it be satisfied by whatever you ate right now (even if that was a bowl of raw vegetables)? Or is the sensation somewhere else? Are you actually feeling this "hunger" in your chest, or your throat, or in your head? Will eating x really make this emotion go away? You might be surprised to find that when you pay true attention to the feeling, it starts to become clear that this is actually another emotion entirely, but your brain has learned to interpret it as hunger.*

3. *Don't be afraid to remind yourself that although you are having thoughts about being hungry, this doesn't mean you have to act upon them immediately. Even "tricking" yourself—saying "I will eat x in ten minutes if I still feel the same way"—can be a powerful strategy to reduce the strength of your desire to eat right now. Just the simple act of paying attention to what your body is trying to tell you may even make the feeling start to disappear. This does, however, mean that you might have to endure the emotion instead of avoiding it, which I know can be painful and challenging. But learning alternative ways to cope with this is the first step to freedom from the vicious cycle of emotional eating.*

Bringing this little moment of awareness to the situation can help to retrain our brains from reading all sorts of different emotional signals simply as hunger. Even if you only remember to do this exercise from time to time, or even just once, it can still be very worthwhile.

RECOGNIZING THE TRIGGERS FOR EMOTIONAL EATING

The next stage might be to explore whether there are certain situations, triggers, or cues that particularly set you off on the path toward emotional eating. Give yourself five minutes each evening to look back over the day and to recognize if there were any times when you emotionally ate. I usually suggest trying this for a week or so, to see if you can find any patterns emerging.

The following table might help you to examine and process those thoughts. Remember, as with all of these exercises, there are no right or wrong answers.

TRIGGER/CUE	Disagreement with partner (trigger)	3 p.m. coffee break at work (cue)
EMOTION	Sadness, rejection, anger	Boredom
PHYSICAL SENSATION	Tight feeling in chest, heart racing	Fatigue
FOOD/EATING REACTION	Ate lots of toast with butter and jam, plus a chocolate bar	Ate two cookies with my coffee
FEELINGS AFTER EATING	Annoyed with myself, felt disgusting and guilty. Low self-esteem thoughts came back strongly.	Felt like I had failed—I'd "blown it" for the day. Ended up having three glasses of wine this evening, which I didn't really want.
WHAT COULD I DO DIFFERENTLY? HOW HAVE I HANDLED THIS BETTER IN THE PAST?	Take some time out to cool off by going for a 15-minute walk, or similar. Work on our communication skills. Maybe I could have handled the situation more constructively.	Be aware that I have a slump at 3 p.m. Make sure my lunch is filling and stabilizes my blood sugars. Have a healthy alternative in my desk in case I am hungry. Try a 5-minute walk before having a cookie.

I define "triggers" as situations you *cannot* predict (such as an argument with your partner, a hurtful comment, a bereavement) and "cues" as situations you *can* predict, which can lead to emotional eating habits (such as walking in through the door after work, the 3 p.m. coffee break, watching TV in the evenings). Both triggers and cues are worth thinking about, however minor they may seem, because they can both precipitate different types of emotional eating. What are your triggers and cues? Have they changed over time?

Your route map out is the last row of the chart opposite. These solutions are not something that any book can tell you or list, because they are so personal. But if this feels like something that resonates with you, I suggest that you dedicate a little bit of time to this exercise before you carry on through the rest of the chapters. If you still find yourself struggling, it might be a good idea to seek out some professional help.

Emotional eating is so very important to work on, because fundamentally food is not the solution to difficult emotions. So the sooner we can find alternative strategies to comfort and console ourselves, the better all round.

A note about emotional snacking . . .

Nourish & Glow: The 10-Day Plan *suggests that you eat three times a day and no more than that. This can be a double-edged sword for people who struggle with emotional eating. On the one hand, it takes away any decisions about whether and what to eat outside of meals, which may be a relief to some. But to others that can seem rather scary; after all, your emotional crutch has also been taken away. However, once you have worked through these exercises, you will have started to come up with all sorts of strategies for alternative options, whereas previously you may have sought comfort from food. Preparation is definitely empowerment.*

Tips for "good mood food"

Our mood can influence the foods we choose, but the foods we eat can influence our emotions too. So how do we create a virtuous cycle of "good mood food"?

1. *Stabilize your blood sugars.*

   Cut down on refined carbohydrates and sugar, creating your meals from whole foods instead, like fresh vegetables and a portion of protein.

2. *Up your omega-3 fats.*

   Try to eat 1–2 portions of oily fish, such as salmon, trout, mackerel, herring, or sardines a week, or consider taking a high-quality fish oil supplement.

3. *Reduce your omega-6 fats.*

   Ditch the sunflower and vegetable oils and processed foods, and cook from scratch with olive oil or coconut oil instead.

4. *Eat polyphenols.*

   Berries, cocoa, green tea and the whole rainbow of fruits and vegetables are great sources of these health-giving compounds. Even a small glass (around 4 oz) of red wine can be beneficial.

5. *Wean yourself off your reliance on caffeine.*

   Too much caffeine can make us feel more tired, rather than less. This feels counterintuitive, but over a long period our bodies adapt to what we give them, so we end up needing caffeine just to feel normal.

6. *Get your B vitamins.*

   Eat plenty of green leafy vegetables, nuts, seeds, and eggs. I encourage whole foods first, but vegans may need to supplement.

7. Boost your fiber.

Our gut microflora (friendly bacteria) are now thought to play an important role in our mood. The best way to give them a boost is to eat a minimally processed, varied, high-fiber diet.

Following the guidelines in this book will help you to optimize all of these without having to think about them too hard.

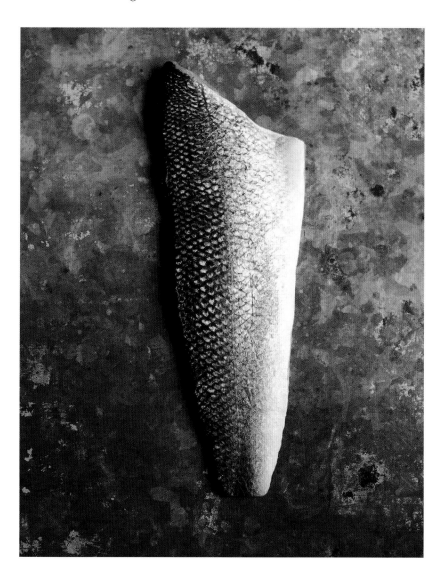

THE WILLPOWER MYTH

Do you consider your willpower to be a finite resource that will run out if you ask too much of it? Well, you're not alone. That is what we have been told time and time again in books, in magazines, and by the wellness community. So although we may stick perfectly to the program all week long, we end up blaming our low willpower reserves if we have a binge on the weekend.

In fact, willpower is something that you can work on, like a muscle. Every time you successfully use your willpower, you are more capable of doing the same next time. So instead of draining your resolve, you are actually topping it up and helping it to grow stronger.

But how you think about your willpower is pretty vital. If you *believe* that you don't have enough of it to stick with your new habits, then that is likely to come true. If instead you believe that you can *develop* your willpower, make it stronger, and even come to rely on it when you are feeling weak, then you are able to put yourself in a far more positive place.

At those times when you are truly struggling—when you just do not think you can stick with it—instead of blaming your willpower, ask yourself what it is you really need right now. What is making this moment so hard? What have you done in the past in situations like this that has been helpful?

It is 3:30 p.m., and someone has put out a plate of homemade cookies in the staff coffee room. You are really struggling to resist—they just look so tempting—but you don't really want to eat any.

Ask yourself what is making this moment so hard.

You feel like you will be missing out, and you feel you deserve a little treat after a hard morning.

What could you do in situations like this instead?

Make a cup of tea and eat a piece of fruit, or head out for a 5-minute walk to break the state.

Here's another way to flex your willpower muscle.

Saying a polite but firm "No" to both yourself and your colleagues. Imagining yourself one hour from now—and feeling really proud that you have stuck to a diet that served and nourished your body. It wasn't a "worth it" moment to go off track with your food choices (as it might be for your own birthday cake or a special dessert at your favorite restaurant).

Willpower is *not* about learning to live a life of deprivation or "white-knuckling" it for the rest of time, always fighting with yourself about whether you should or shouldn't eat something. That sounds utterly exhausting and rather miserable, if you ask me! Willpower is there to be on your side, and to help support you (especially at the beginning of any new lifestyle change, when new habits haven't been formed yet and old ones are still making their way out the door) until you are able to do it with genuine ease and joy.

THIS IS YOUR EXISTENCE

This profound concept has brought an enormous shift in my own consciousness and that of my clients, and I want to share it with you.

It sounds strange to have to spell it out, because of course we all *know* that this is our life, but it amazes me how many people are almost "putting off" living it fully because of their low self-esteem. It is as if they are living in a period of suspended animation, waiting to get going again just as soon as they feel better about themselves (which is often linked to an arbitrary weight goal or dress size).

If you are being truly honest with yourself, how often do you have thoughts similar to these?

- "If only I was slimmer."
- "I am not going to wear/do x looking like this."
- "When I reach x weight, I will do it/go there/be happy."
- "Life will be better once I am healthier/thinner/fitter."
- "I don't deserve to have x if I feel like this."

People are often on this yo-yo diet bandwagon for the majority of their adult lives, and so many decades of their existence are marred by critical and withholding thoughts. They are simply unable to lead their fullest life because of food. *It should not be like this.*

But this, right now—every second, every minute, every day—is your life. It is *not* a period of suspended animation, and one thing is for certain: you're only going to get one shot at it. You are already *living your existence.* So is this the existence you wanted? Or is it one that is excessively influenced, or even controlled, by food and your thoughts around it?

"We are what we think about all day long."

—Ralph Waldo Emerson

Remember that you absolutely have a choice. You can *choose* instead to embrace each day and its opportunities, to learn grace and perspective around food, and to work toward a point where food is working *for* you, not against you.

Give yourself some space to think about it, if you think that might be helpful. Even reach out and ask those around you for support if necessary.

But whatever you do, please decide that from this moment on you will let go of that burden of criticism you are carrying around. And remember to say to yourself *this is my existence* when that negative self-doubt tries to hold you back.

When thinking about what we eat gets a little out of control

I have seen many clients in my practice over the years who have struggled with disordered eating, in a variety of forms. Eating disorders are a complex and highly personal mixture of behaviors and experiences, and individual situations can vary dramatically. Unfortunately, it is beyond the scope of this book to try to tackle such issues, but if you are worried, I wholeheartedly encourage you to seek appropriate professional help, and I wish you the very best of luck on your journey.

MOVING FORWARD

I hope that this chapter has encouraged you think about what, how, why and with whom you eat—and the implications this has on your ability to make healthy choices around food. We are all unique when it comes to food culture and mind-set, and yet it is exactly this psychology that can be the difference between long-term success and yet another "diet" that you give up on a couple of weeks down the line.

Now that we have started to clear away a little of the historical "baggage" we may have around food and eating, it's time to move into a new way of thinking. I hope it is going to be more practical, less intertwined with emotions, and much, much more positive.

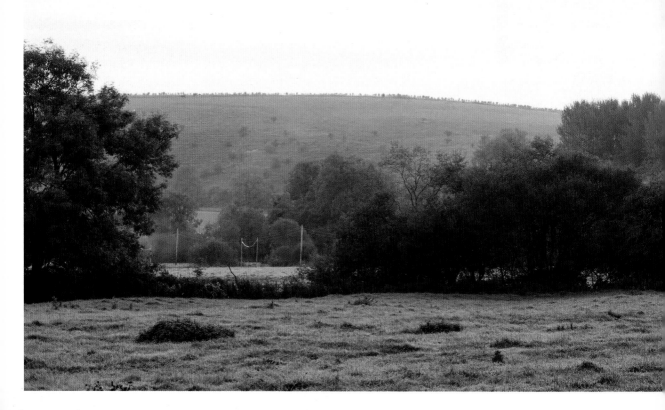

*"Choose to be optimistic
and believe in yourself.
It makes change so
much easier to achieve."*

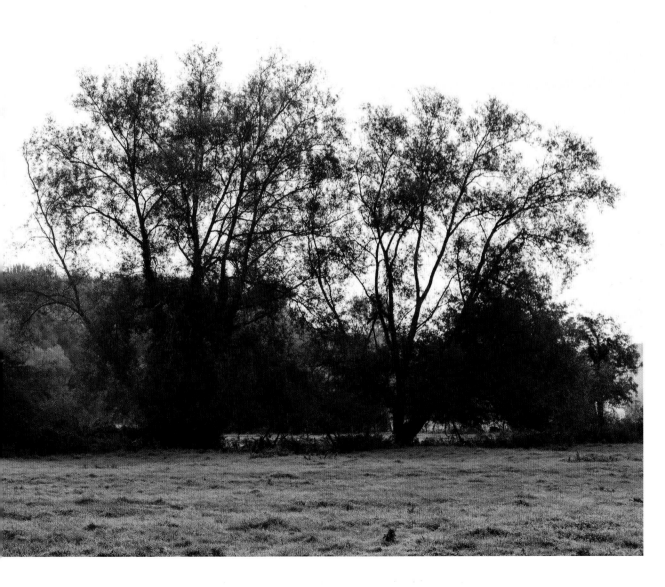

Chapter Two:
BUILDING THE FOUNDATIONS

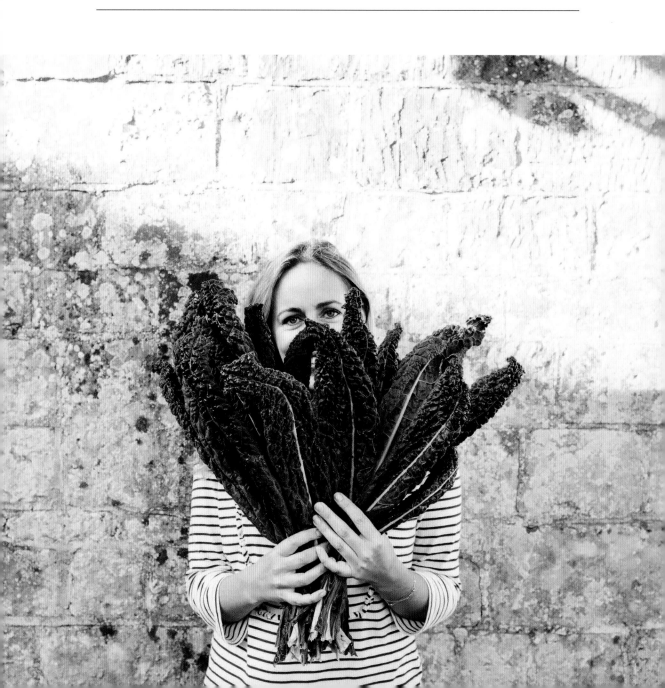

Now it's time to start thinking about how to build strong foundations to support moving forward toward change.

I like to think about this in two ways:

1. *Building up and securing our psychological foundations*
2. *Ensuring that our practical foundations are laid*

There are many things that we can do to make sure that any changes we make "stick," and to avoid falling off the wagon after a few weeks when the novelty has started to wear off. And that starts with understanding why we are trying to make a change in the first place.

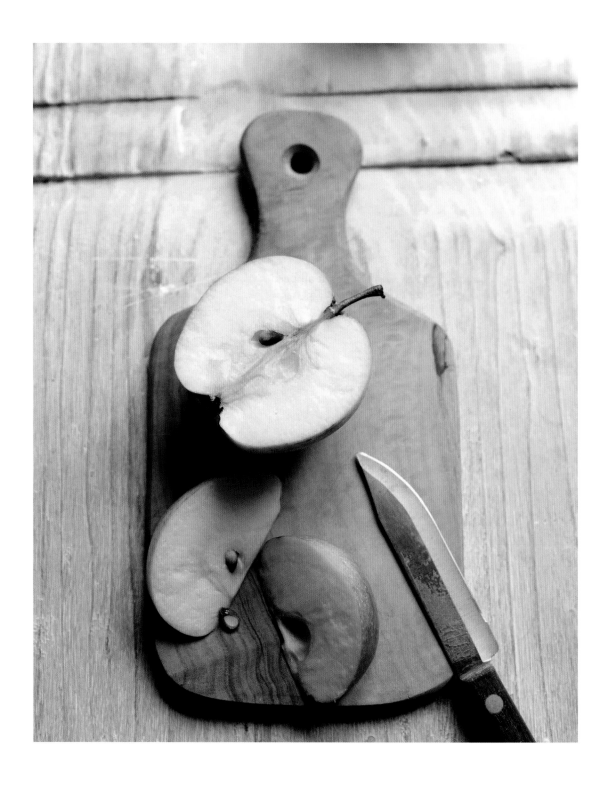

FINDING YOUR CORE REASONS

I don't know about you, but I find it hard to make lifestyle changes (especially in the early days when it all feels quite strange) without really knowing *why* I am doing it. I need to have the end in mind at the start. Making changes is hard—there is no doubt about that. That's because our brain has to work flat-out to learn all of those new skills and habits and all of that knowledge. However, just like when we learn to ride a bike or drive a car, soon enough it all becomes almost automatic, and the change no longer needs so much effort. So although it can be really tough sometimes, it is, without doubt, completely worthwhile and it does get easier, I promise.

Well-established research tells us that people are often more motivated to avoid pain than they are to seek pleasure. However, if we start out on a lifestyle change only because we are trying to "get away" from negative feelings, such as health worries, anxieties over body weight, fear, and confusion, we risk losing our motivation.

This is because as we start to succeed, perhaps losing a few pounds or eating more healthily, our motivation to maintain it can then *decrease*. The fears, the things we are trying to get away from, can start to shrink too.

We can prepare ourselves for this by focusing on, and understanding, the positive reasons *why* we are putting in such an effort, and what our goals are. This makes it all much easier to stick with it when the going gets tough.

Most of us have one or two primary reasons for trying to lead a healthier life. These are the "headline" titles. Things like "because I want to see my kids grow up," "to look drop-dead gorgeous in my wedding dress," "to boost my sports performance." What are yours? I suggest you write them down. If they have a negative slant, can you transform them into the positive? So instead of writing, for example, "to stop getting any sicker," write "to support my body back to full health."

Try to be as open and honest with yourself as you can. If possible, write down absolutely everything that comes into your head, as the act of seeing it in black and white on paper can be so helpful. Nobody else need ever read it.

For years my list turned out to be based on meeting other people's expectations, and it has been wonderful for me to shed that list and instead flip my goals to meet my own needs, and indeed learn what my needs actually are.

Keep your list close (take a photo of it to keep on your phone) and in moments when you are struggling to stick with your new habits, take a quick look at it to remind yourself why you started this journey in the first place.

If at any point throughout this book you find you have dug up some surprisingly strong emotions and are not sure how to cope with them, I urge you to seek out some support from either a close friend, a family member, or a qualified health professional. Our relationship with food is often deeply linked to our core emotions and memories, and sometimes when we examine these closely it can feel like a bit of a tangled mess with no clear route out. Do not be afraid to reach out for help. It is not a sign of weakness and is far better than trying to work it all out alone.

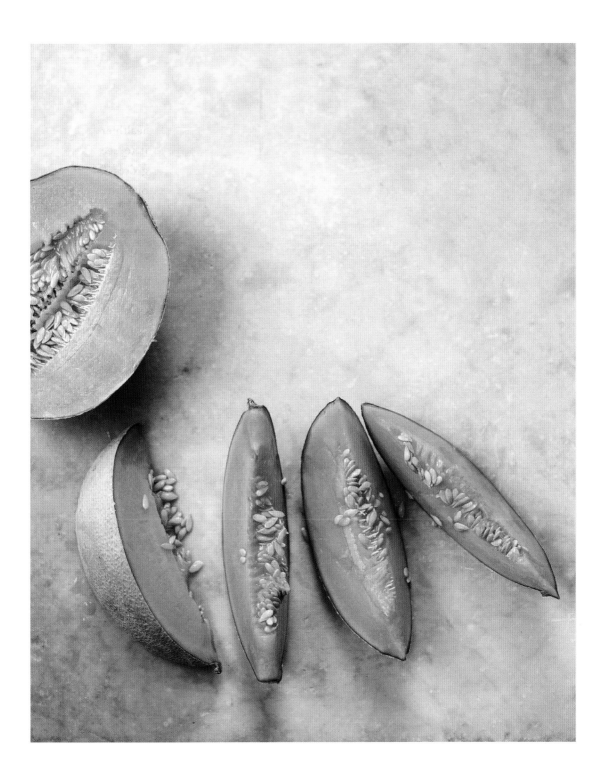

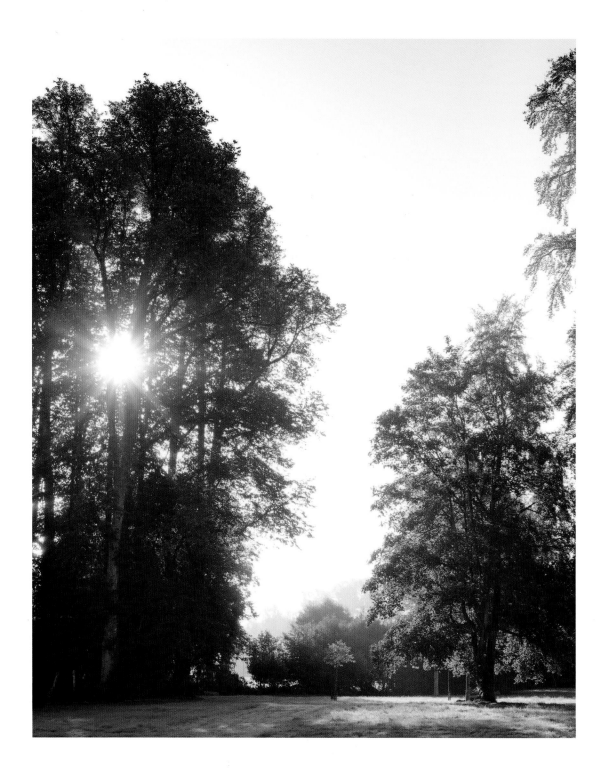

VISUALIZING THE FUTURE YOU

Mindful Exercise

This visualization exercise will help you to create a clear and motivating picture of where you are heading. In a moment of quiet, take a few minutes to really concentrate on the following questions. Imagine exactly what it will *feel* like, what it will *look* like, *sound* like, even *taste* and *smell* like. Bring brightly colored, immersive pictures into your mind, and grow them as large as possible. Really embrace the image and make that positive future a part of you.

1. *What will it be like when you have made these changes? Imagine your future self glowing with health and happiness, and allow it to become very clear in your mind exactly what that will be like.*

2. *What will you be doing that is different? Try thinking through an imaginary day in the future, from the moment you wake up to the moment you go to bed. What does your imaginary future daily routine involve?*

3. *How do you feel as you imagine this future day as your future self?*

4. *What are the steps that you will take to reach your positive future self? Visualize each step, breaking down the whole wellness journey into manageable chunks. Try to really picture what each step will feel like as it is completed.*

Any time you are feeling downhearted, worried that it isn't working, or tempted to step off the wagon, try to bring yourself back to this visualization. Remember, your future self will most certainly thank you for staying the course once you have become that person for real.

FAST VERSUS SLOW CHANGE

Next, we need to transform that list of core reasons into habits and actions.

I recently read a brilliant book called *Better than Before* by Gretchen Rubin. It really helped me to understand how and why we form habits—and what this means for any lifestyle transformation in the long term. The principles in this section are inspired by Gretchen's work.

I think there are two main ways to go about making changes to your diet, and there is certainly a time and a place for both. The first is the all-or-nothing approach. This is particularly useful if you are, for example, suffering from symptoms that you feel might be food-related and you want to give a strict elimination diet a try. However, you may wish to talk this through with a qualified professional first.

There is a great analogy to explain this all-in approach, which I often use with my clients: If you accidentally step on two thumbtacks, removing just one pin won't make the discomfort go away, because the other one is still sending pain signals to your brain. You need to remove both the tacks to allow yourself to recover. It is the same with certain dietary changes. You need to remove all the potentially triggering foods to allow your gut and your body to recover and start to feel the benefits.

There are other reasons to give the all-in change a try too. Sometimes when we try something radical (even if it is only for a short period of time) it throws a little perspective on to our usual habits and can hit "refresh" on our mind-set. We may become more aware of our unconscious actions, or feel more empowered to stick with a few less extreme changes in the future. It's the "if I can do *that*, then I can do *anything*" feeling most of us have experienced at some point or other.

There are lots of people, however, who find that these kind of extreme changes are overly restricting and just make them want to rebel.

The second way to make dietary changes is the stepwise approach. This can be a great way to sustain a number of new health habits in the longer term. We are often better at making one small change at a time, allowing it to become gradually ingrained in our everyday lives, than making lots of changes all at once. This goes against the instant-gratification culture that we find ourselves in, with magazine covers promoting diets that will supposedly help us lose "ten pounds in ten days" or transform us into "bikini-body models in six weeks."

Tempting promises, admittedly! But the problem is that sadly it just doesn't work. Study after study has shown that crash diets not only cause us to lose mainly water weight (especially over the first few days), but may also lead to changes in our metabolism that can last long after we put the weight back on. We all know people (maybe even ourselves) who seem to have tried every diet under the sun without long-term success, even with the most radical of approaches.

So, you may wish to do a really strict elimination diet or take a slow approach by doing one thing at a time. As the middle ground, the 10-day plan in this book has been created to be flexible enough to let you decide. For example, you can follow it to the letter for ten days or you can choose to just start with the breakfasts—there really is no right or wrong way.

"Patience is not the ability to wait, but how you act while you're waiting."

—Joyce Meyer

WHY DO AN ELIMINATION DIET?

Our bodies have evolved over thousands of years to work best on a broad and varied diet that changes with the seasons. It seems sensible, therefore, that we should still try to eat as wide a range of foods as we can, so that we have access to the greatest array of nutrients possible. Even different varieties of the same fruit or vegetable, for example, will have slightly different nutritional profiles and benefits.

I suppose all this diversity is also a way of hedging our bets against nutritional imbalances, striking a happy medium between underconsuming certain foods on the one hand, and overconsuming foods on the other. According to this theory, then, the more dietary limits we put on ourselves, whether by choice, by habit, or by necessity, the harder it will be for us to reach a state of optimal nutrition.

So why purposefully go on an elimination diet? The very nature of it seems to go against our need to eat as varied a diet as possible.

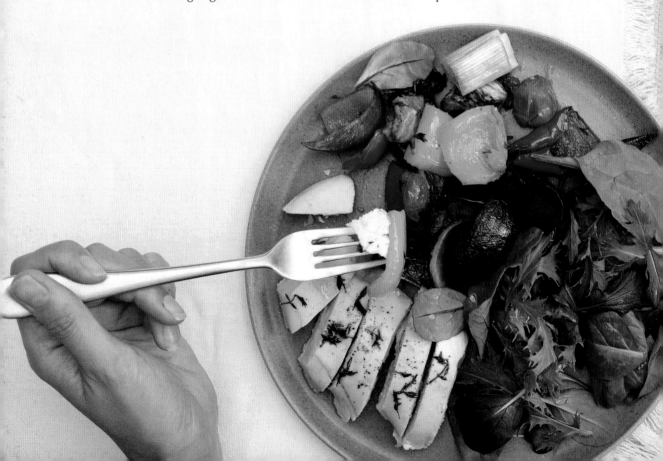

I think that there are probably four reasons why people choose to undertake an elimination-type diet:

1. A basic elimination diet

   (somewhat counterintuitively) can actually increase the variety of foods you eat (see next page for an explanation). I hope that this is how you feel if you complete the 10-day meal plan.

2. It is a diet free from processed and junk food,

   with a lot more emphasis on plenty of fresh produce and whole foods.

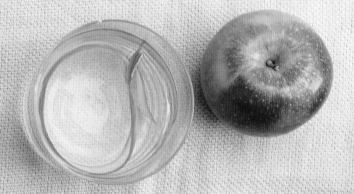

3. Moving away from our typical, often automatic routine

   can bring a little more mindfulness and consciousness to our food choices and eating habits—which can continue long after the elimination part of the diet has stopped.

4. Food sensitivities and intolerances may be an overlooked cause of nagging (or sometimes even severe) symptons.

   An elimination diet may play a useful role in helping you to manage these, although it is important to speak to your doctor or another health professional first, to make sure you are not missing anything more serious.

You might be surprised that by cutting out (or down on) certain food groups that you have come to rely upon, you may actually *increase* the variety of foods that you eat.

An average day of food for someone who is fairly health conscious:

- Breakfast: **Wheat cereal** with a chopped banana and **semi-skimmed milk. Latte.**

- Lunch: **Whole-grain bread**, organic **cheese** and lettuce sandwich, apple, and some carrot sticks. Glasses of water.

- Supper: **Brown pasta** with homemade tomato sauce, big green salad, and **grated Parmesan**.

But let's look a little closer. All three meals are predominantly made up of processed **wheat** of some kind or another (cereal, bread, pasta), or **milk-based dairy** products (milk or cheese). In fact, these two main ingredients are making up the bulk of the food energy for the day. Only a handful of other foods are being consumed. Therefore, by removing wheat and dairy products, this person would be encouraged to seek alternative options. This may actually broaden their dietary intake by eating more fruits, vegetables, nuts, protein sources, etc.

A typical basic elimination day:

- Breakfast: Gluten-free overnight oats with seeds, nut milk, and chopped banana.

- Lunch: Big salad with carrot sticks, cucumber, lettuce leaves, hummus, sweet corn, beets, seeds, and an apple.

- Supper: Zucchini "noodles" with homemade tomato sauce, grilled chicken breast, and a big green salad drizzled with extra-virgin olive oil. A handful of blueberries.

The more you eliminate, however, the less likely this counterintuitive increase in variety is likely to happen, and the risk of nutritional imbalances increases (not to mention the increased anxiety that can come from imposing an unnecessarily restrictive diet on yourself). There is a happy medium!

And while they have been highlighted in these examples, wheat and dairy are not "bad" for you (in most circumstances). Indeed, they contain a variety of beneficial nutrients and can absolutely be part of a healthy diet. However, I have excluded them from the 10-day plan for a couple of reasons. One is that this allows us the opportunity to try out all sorts of new ingredients and dishes instead, and the other is that I wanted to demonstrate what a healthy gluten-free diet, specifically, might look like (enjoying naturally gluten-free foods, rather than relying on the processed "free-from" versions). There is no harm in giving this a try, and you can always reintroduce both gluten and dairy again if you want to at the end of the plan.

As with all major nutritional changes, it is important to ask a qualified nutrition professional to guide you through this process if you are planning to eat a restrictive diet beyond a few days or so.

A note on intolerances and allergies:

We now know that "one size" can *never* "fit all," however good a nutrition plan might be. That goes for this book too! If you are someone who suffers from an intolerance, or from allergies, you may find that the 10-day plan is difficult for you to follow to the letter. Just make any adjustments you need to, or indeed pick and choose any recipes that you can enjoy.

Other types of elimination diets:

There are a lot of different terms used to describe elimination diets (which just means that certain foods, or food groups, are excluded), so I thought it might be helpful to outline what some of these actually mean. This is not to say that I necessarily advocate them, but I do believe that knowing about them is useful in helping us to understand nutrition in a wider context—and also to help protect us against all that pesky marketing!

TYPES OF ELIMINATION DIETS

Almost all healthy diets, whether they are elimination diets or not, would benefit from reducing intake of processed and junk foods, refined carbohydrates (including sugar) and trans fats. As a rule, every type of elimination diet excludes all of these foods as a baseline.

1. A basic elimination diet also removes gluten and dairy products, as I have done in the 10-day meal plan.

    Many people may then be able to reintroduce one, or both, of these ingredients with no change in how they feel after the period of elimination. They can then continue to enjoy dairy and/or gluten in moderation going forwards. Sufferers of celiac disease, however, need to remain gluten-free for life to manage their condition.

2. A full elimination diet may sometimes be suggested

    (best done under the guidance of a professional), which would also exclude eggs, shellfish, soy and soy products, corn, and tree nuts. Sometimes this is used to diagnose or manage food intolerances, but again, it is important that foods are reintroduced in a systematic manner so that the diet can be as broad and varied as possible.

3. Nightshade (solanaceae) elimination diets exclude products from the nightshade family.

    These include white potatoes, eggplant, tomatoes and tomatillos, goji berries, bell peppers, paprika, and chili peppers. The evidence for doing this diet is not certain, and as many of these foods have health benefits, excluding them *unnecessarily* may not be ideal.

4. The Specific Carbohydrate Diet.

    This is a very restrictive elimination that excludes all grains, certain legumes (soy beans, chickpeas, mung beans, broad beans, and bean sprouts), most dairy products, starches and root vegetables, and canned or processed meats or vegetables. It is hypothesized that this diet helps people with digestive troubles by removing carbohydrates that are reportedly harder to digest. However, by cutting out whole food groups like this, you are also cutting out a vast amount of beneficial nutrition. It should not be undertaken without close nutritional support and the advice of your doctor.

5. The Paleo diet is also an elimination diet of sorts.

It excludes beans, grains, dairy, sugar, and seed oils (eating lots of meat, fish, fruit, vegetables, eggs, nuts and seeds, and other fats like avocado and olive oil instead). Some variations of Paleo (also known as the "primal" diet) include fermented dairy products (like yogurt) and occasional traditional grains.

6. The FODMAP diet.

FODMAPs are fermentable carbohydrates, found in a range of foods, that can be poorly absorbed by some people and can therefore cause digestive issues. The diet is used by dietitians with good effect for people suffering from irritable bowel syndrome. However, staying strictly low-FODMAP for the long term is too restrictive of beneficial nutrients. It should only be undertaken with experienced support.

7. A ketogenic diet may be used by health practitioners to help treat neurological problems like epilepsy.

A ketogenic diet gets around 70 percent of calories from fat, 25 percent from protein and only 5 percent from carbohydrates. This means that almost all forms of carbohydrates are excluded. It should only ever be undertaken with experienced medical or dietetic support, as there can be significant risks, both when starting the diet and while maintaining it.

If I am serious about wanting to make a lifestyle change, I like to ask myself whether I think I could stick with it in a year's time? If not, why not? Is it too unrealistic, too dramatic, too expensive? Is there anything I could do to make the change a little easier to manage?

So let's think what it would be like if we dropped the race-to-the-finish-line approach completely and just accepted that if we want to make sustainable changes for the good of our long-term health then we need to be realistic. What if we decided to choose just one new habit a week, giving ourselves plenty of time to become familiar with it and to tweak it to fit seamlessly into our own life? And only when we are completely happy with the first habit would we move on to the next one. Changing habits one by one is much less overwhelming than trying to change everything at once.

Here are some examples of what those individual habits might look like:

- Including a portion of protein with every breakfast
- Having one more serving of green leafy vegetables each day
- Swapping store-bought dressings for extra-virgin olive oil and lemon juice
- Drinking a large glass of water half an hour before each meal
- Eating only when sitting down

Whichever route to habit change you choose, remember that you can go completely at your own pace—this is not race. There is no finish line.

Case study: Radical Diets

I was asked for help by a male client who had struggled with his weight from a young age. A few years before seeing me, he had been told by his doctor that he had developed prediabetic changes, and this spurred him into a really radical lifestyle overhaul. He had read about a new diet that promised spectacular results and decided to give it a try. The only catch? He couldn't eat. At all. The only nutrition to pass his lips was in the form of food-supplement drinks. And, extraordinarily, he stuck to it religiously for twelve months. Not one piece of food passed his lips in all that time. And the results were dramatic—he lost almost seventy pounds.

But the moment he stopped using the drinks, the weight started to pile back on. His metabolism had been affected by the long-term semistarvation that it had been subjected to, and so eating even a moderate diet was causing significant weight gain. By the time I saw him, all of the weight was back on, plus a little extra. And why? Because not one of his old habits had actually been changed sustainably during those 12 months. So, we started again—and this time used a far more realistic stepwise approach. One habit change a week. One day at a time. And slowly but surely he is losing all of that weight again. But this time he is also managing to keep it off.

THE STEPWISE APPROACH:
choosing your habits

If you are ready to get going, a great place to start is by writing down a list of new habits you would like to adopt.

It can be helpful to think about them under the following five category headings:

1. *How I plan and think about my food*

   (e.g., planning menus, working on mind-set)

2. *How I shop for my food*

   (e.g., having fresh vegetables available, not buying cookies)

3. *How I cook and prepare my food*

   (e.g., taking lunch to work, Sunday prep day)

4. *How I eat and drink*

   (e.g., mindful eating, moderate alcohol intake, plenty of water, etc.)

5. *Other ways to improve my lifestyle*

   (e.g., exercise, sleep, stress, smoking)

As you write down these new habits, try to ensure that they are highly specific, positive (i.e., what you *will* do rather than what you *won't* do), and related to the *behaviors or actions* that will help you to fulfill your reasons for making a change, rather than to the reasons themselves.

TIP: It is often better to start by adding in healthy habits than by taking away less healthy ones. That can come later, when we do not necessarily want or need them so much any more.

Building the Foundations

- ✎ "I will walk 10,000 steps a day, at least six days a week" rather than "I will exercise more"

- ✎ "I will drink three glasses of water before lunchtime each day" rather than "I will drink more"

- ✎ "I will eat a portion of nuts and seeds every day" rather than "I will not eat chocolate cookies"

- ✎ "I will make myself a packed lunch four days this week" rather than "I will stop buying lunch at work"

Once you have come up with your list of habits, ask yourself how confident you are, out of 5 (with 1 being very unsure and 5 being extremely confident), that you can maintain each change, every day, over the next month. If your honest answer is less than 4 or 5, then you need to adjust the habit so that it is easier. You are aiming for your answer to this question to be: "Of course I can do that—it's so ridiculously easy!"

It is often better to make a tiny change that you can stick to than to make a bigger change that only lasts a couple of days. There is no shame in your changes being small, if that means they are more achievable. You have complete control over how easy or hard a new habit is, so why not start off easy? You can make them more challenging if you want to in the future.

TIP: Focus on the pleasure or the benefits (such as the time or money you are saving) that those changes could bring you. Personally, I focus on having better energy and skin!

TIP: One of the best ways to help yourself stick with a new habit is to keep a very simple record. I draw a little square in the top page of my diary for that day, and tick it when I have completed my habit. Or you can set a phone reminder.

CREATING YOUR COMMUNITY

Finding a like-minded person (or people) that we can share our experiences and progress with can really help motivate us and boost our chances of long-term success. Having someone to lean on for support and motivation, to highlight our excuses or when we put things off, is key. They can also help hold us accountable for our choices and guide us back on track if we find ourselves straying a little. This person doesn't necessarily need to be going through a lifestyle transformation themselves, but they do need to be willing and able to support our journey without becoming the food police.

They could be a friend, family member, colleague, even an older child (it's amazing how children notice if you don't do something you've said you would!), or something a little more structured—such as a support group, doctor, nutritionist, or personal trainer. The key is to find a person or people you trust, respect, and feel able to be honest with. Share your expectations openly from the outset, and decide how often you are going to "check in." This will depend entirely on your individual schedules, but I suggest that a quick update every other day by text is a good starting point, perhaps meeting face to face once every 1–2 weeks. As your journey progresses, you may find that you need less frequent check-ins.

You can also use social media to your advantage here. As I covered in Chapter One, the more we surround ourselves with other people who are leading a healthy lifestyle, the more likely we are to stick to a healthy lifestyle ourselves. Go through your social media accounts and unfollow anything that no longer serves you, makes you feel bad about yourself, or just offers unhelpful temptations.

And perhaps transform your social media platforms into places of positive motivation—where the online community will support and inspire you, and buoy you up when you're having a bad day. But try to be a little skeptical when creating your social media community—if a lifestyle or body looks too good to be true, it more than likely is.

Tips for creating your support community

1. Practical support

Think about practical ways your friends and family can support your changes. Maybe someone could watch the kids for an hour while you go for a walk or a jog, or cook plenty of vegetables if you are sharing a meal together. Creating a list can bring a great deal of clarity both for yourself and for those around you.

2. Start a "lunch club" at work

Get together with some of your work colleagues who would also like to eat well at the office, and take turns bringing in lunch for each other. This cuts down on your prep time and is also a fun way to try new recipes.

3. Having fun

Research local activities you can do with friends or family that do not involve just eating and/or drinking. Having a supply of healthy alternatives ready at the drop of a hat can be really helpful when people are wondering what to do together.

4. Speak to the kids

Explain that you want to make some healthy changes and that there will be all sorts of exciting things that you can learn together, as a family, by doing so. Try to frame the reasons for such changes in simple, positive terms that they can relate to: more energy for running and playing, for example. This will help them understand and reduce the anxiety caused by any changes.

5. Find a brand-new community

Joining a fitness class, new club, or support group can be a great way to boost your motivation, particularly in the early stages.

6. Remember the positives

What benefits will your lifestyle changes bring to those around you? Focusing on, and sharing, the good things is a lovely way to garner support.

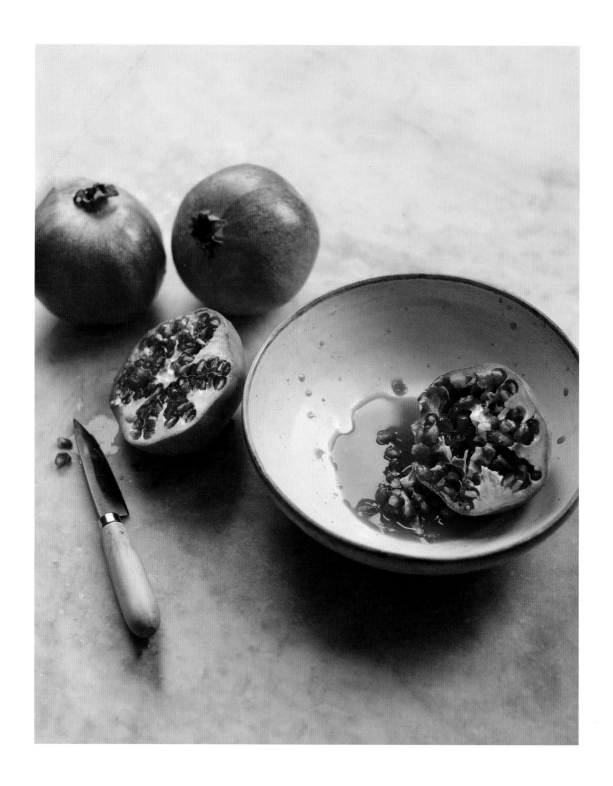

HOW OTHERS MAY "SABOTAGE" YOUR EFFORTS

This is a tricky subject to tackle, because it can really touch a nerve, but I think it is still an important topic to cover because it can, ultimately, be the difference between transformational success and transformational stalemate.

Some, a little, or even none of this may be relevant in your life. If the last part is true, that is wonderful, but I encourage you to read through this section anyway, as understanding these factors can help us to understand the health lives of others with a little more empathy. If the first part is true, perhaps you have experienced a degree of interference from others in previous efforts to change your lifestyle, which have hindered or even undermined your progress altogether. It is an emotionally charged topic, so I will try my hardest to tread carefully!

As discussed in Chapter One, sometimes we use food for emotional purposes that may run much deeper than the everyday tasks of cooking or eating. Perhaps those around you show you their love and affection through giving you food. It can therefore feel rather like a personal attack, a rejection of love, if you refuse it. This can lead to resentment, disappointment, even anger.

Or perhaps you are the primary cook in the household, and nobody else is on board with your ideas for healthier meals (there may even be a few tantrums about it), but you don't have time to cook separate meals every evening.

And what if your key social time normally comes alongside food or alcohol? Whether that's Friday night in the bar or a hungover fried-food brunch on Sundays, sometimes the majority of our downtime with friends or family revolves around consuming things that you are trying to avoid for now. If you find it hard to resist in front of your friends, or you are subject to peer pressure if you do politely refuse, then how are you going to continue seeing them while still supporting your own healthy changes?

Finally, although you may mentally be in the right place to go about making a significant change, your partner or family may not be. Of course, this can be hard to accept, because you desperately want them to get healthy, too, and live long and fulfilling lives. But however much pleading, coercion, or persuasion you use, it really is a thankless task to force someone into changes they do not want to make. Sometimes, however, seeing your positive changes can be the boost that they need to jump aboard too, or perhaps it seems less scary if you do it together.

Given all of these emotionally charged feelings, sadly sometimes people may go so far as to actually sabotage your newfound habits and effort. Perhaps it makes them uncomfortable to see you making the positive changes they know, deep down, that they should really be making too; perhaps they just dislike change altogether; or perhaps they are worried that your relationship may also change. I have seen many a client stumble when this problem arises. So if this is you, then do not feel alone. I do not really believe that most people behaving like this are actively trying to be unkind; it is far more a reflection of their own thoughts and feelings around relationships and food than it is of them as a person.

We all need connections—our families, friends, partners, and colleagues—in our lives, but it's important to feel supported and encouraged.

In order to address this problem, first we need to understand it. Taking a moment to step into the other person's shoes (however uncomfortable or angry that makes you feel) can be a very helpful step toward resolving the conflict.

So here are some of the common underlying fears and reactions I have come across, as well as some strategies to help everyone to work through them. This is by no means an exhaustive list, but I hope that it gives you a few helpful ideas nonetheless.

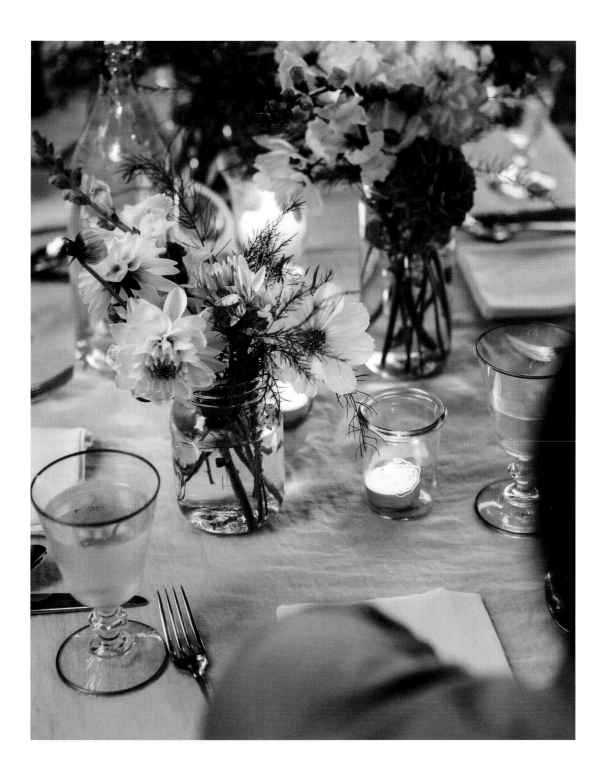

COMMON "SABOTAGE"	EXAMPLE PHRASE	COPING STRATEGIES
Temptation	"Go on . . . one little slice isn't going to hurt, is it? You deserve it."	Usually a firm polite, "Not today, thanks" works well for this one. Sometimes you need to repeat it a few times!
Creating guilt	"You're just making us all look bad, aren't you?"	Sometimes laughing this one off is the best bet, but you could also just say that you are doing it for your own personal reasons.
Undermining your willpower and effort	"I've cooked you your favorite cake as a special treat. I can't wait to see you try some!"	Prior explanations may help you avoid this situation, but if someone has done it knowingly, then have a calm conversation (maybe another time) to help them understand why.
Health worries	"You are losing too much weight— you'll soon waste away."	Reassurance that this is no crash diet, that you know what a healthy weight is, and that you have no intention of going below this. Explain your changes as a dietary "upgrade" rather than any sort of deprivation.
Nostalgia	"But I like the 'old' you. Why do you want to change?"	This reaction often comes from a love—but it may come from associating the "old" you with comfort and indulgence, which they now miss. Perhaps you feel able to share your "core reasons" list—and show that this is not just some phase. Discuss specific worries and offer reassurance that this you is still you.

COMMON "SABOTAGE"	EXAMPLE PHRASE	COPING STRATEGIES
Special occasions	"Oh, won't you even just have one more? It's Halloween/ a holiday/Great-aunt Maud's birthday!"	Sometimes it really is "worth it," in which case, embrace the moment with full enjoyment, but try to politely stick to your guns when it's not.
Feeling rejected	"But you love my lasagna. What's wrong with it now?"	Having a chat ahead of time can sometimes avoid this awkward situation. Thank them for their kindness, but reiterate that this is nothing to do with their cooking; it is just that you are trying to stick to a healthy diet.
Self-reflection or low self-esteem	(Often unspoken) "Now you've made all these changes, it makes me feel even worse about my own lifestyle/weight."	Non-judgment is key, as is avoiding making comparisons between your new lifestyle and your loved ones' current choices. Remain open to help, but only if they specifically ask for it.
Unwanted gifts	"I've ordered your favorite takeout so you don't need to cook now." "Here's a box of your favorite chocolates."	Thank them for the kind thought, but ask for their help in the future to stick to your own diet/program. Maybe have a small portion, and pile up veggies on the side. Share or donate any unwanted food presents.
Discouragement	"Don't you know that diets never work? You won't be able to keep it up." "Everyone puts the weight back on eventually."	Explain that this is not a diet, it is simply healthy eating, and you are really proud of your efforts so far.

Tips to prevent sabotage

What else can we do to help stop lifestyle "sabotage" from ruining our goals?

1. Be realistic.

Find those who are on board with your changes and lean on them if possible, but you can still continue to pursue your goals without the wholehearted support of everyone around you.

2. Explain yourself to those you feel might create resistance.

Find a few quiet moments to explain that you have decided to make some changes to your diet and lifestyle for the benefit of your own long-term health. This is not something that you feel is negotiable; it is a firm decision that you have come to after a lot of thought. Tell them that you would be very grateful for their support, as you know it won't always be easy, so knowing they are there for you would be an enormous help. Go on to reassure them that this is no fad or silly diet and that there is always going to be room for the odd slice of birthday cake! Allow space for the other person/people to raise any concerns they may have about your plans. Addressing these calmly from the outset smooths out a lot of worry further down the line. Issues may be raised that you never would have thought of.

3. Get people involved.

Kids not so sure about the new food? Try getting them to help you with the shopping or food preparation. Browse online or in books and choose recipes together. Perhaps you could even ask them to devise their own special three-course "healthy menu" that you will cook together one weekend. Explore new ingredients and flavors together— and reassure them that most people, even adults, don't like things the first time they try them (our bodies naturally reject new tastes in case they are dangerous), but sticking at it and trying them ten times usually transforms a dislike into a like. Friends reluctant healthy eaters? Prepare a dinner party for them, to showcase your favorite new dishes. Whatever it is, involving people in your journey encourages them to feel more invested in your success—and the more invested people feel, the more strongly they will be able to support you.

4. Believe in yourself.

There are ups and downs in every transformation, but staying persistent is critical to your long-term success. When people have seen you stick to your guns a few times, they will often stop trying to sabotage you at all. Keep reading your list of true reasons if you find that your enthusiasm is starting to fade. Remember that you have within you the ability to transform, so flex that willpower muscle and make it even stronger. Don't forget that you are an adult, so what goes in your mouth, how often you exercise, or how you react to those emotional trip hazards is your responsibility, but that also means it is within your power to change.

5. Don't sabotage yourself!

Perhaps you recognize that it is, in fact, yourself more than anyone else who is employing these "sabotage" tactics? If this is the case, then keeping a diary can be helpful to show how such thoughts are impacting on your personal diet or health actions. Can you work out why you are doing this? Sometimes it can be easier to fully understand yourself through discussion with a trained professional—perhaps a counselor, or in a group setting. You should feel absolutely no shame in asking for help with these issues. Think of it instead as a proactive step, just like clearing out your cupboards of junk food or buying yourself a new pair of running shoes.

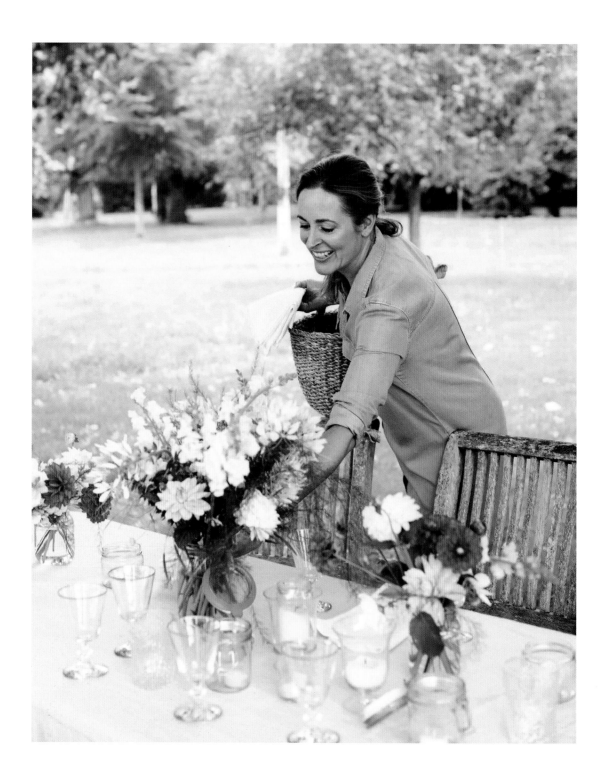

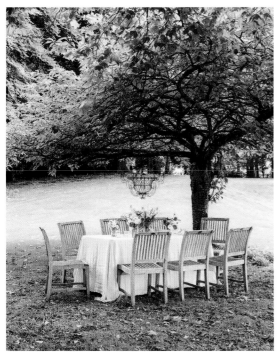

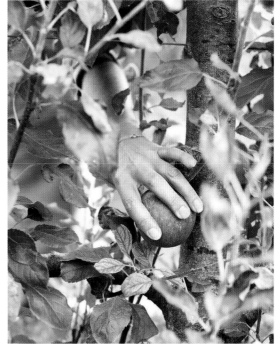

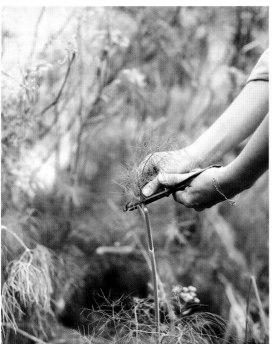

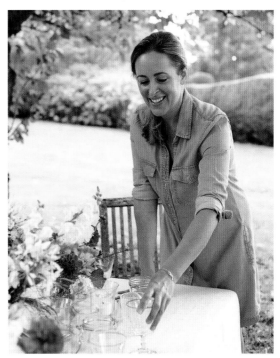

THERE IS NO SUCH THING AS FAILURE

We all hold quite concrete thoughts about what is "right" and what is "wrong." These have helped us to navigate the world safely, to be socially appropriate, to make a career, and much more. But when it comes to diet, these two words, and the concrete thinking behind them, can be rather unhelpful.

That is because all food sits somewhere in a misty, murky shade of gray between "right" and "wrong."

Yes, some foods are less healthy than others. Yes, some days we eat more than other days. But neither option is rigidly "right" or "wrong." Letting go of these labels means that we can show ourselves a little compassion if we don't stick 100 percent to the plan, and if we don't reach our goals in the time frame that we set, then we do not consider that we have "failed"—or, even worse, that we are a failure.

Nobody can be perfect all of the time—and aiming for unrealistic expectations can make us feel like we are constantly striving for the mythical "end of the rainbow"—it is always out of reach, we are always falling a little short. Fighting against those feelings of inadequacy at the same time as trying to stay positive and enthusiastic about the changes we are making is like pushing a boulder up a mountain path. So let's make it easier for ourselves, and leave that boulder behind. This is harder for some than it is for others (myself included—I can be a real perfectionist!), but for those who needed to hear it, these words will have resonated.

"Be gentle with yourself.
You're doing the best you can."

Accepting from the beginning that perfection is impossible will help to prevent catastrophic thinking if something happens that we hoped to avoid—and it will, because that is life. When this does happen, whatever form it may take, you have not failed in any way. So there is no need to throw in the towel and give up on the entire day/weekend/week because of one slip-up. Nor is there any need to punish yourself by cutting back on meals or exercising more in the future. Accept it for what it is—just another shade of gray—and guide yourself gently back onto the path. If you find this happening a lot, then instead of pushing against it harder, take a breather. Why is it happening? Is there something else going on? What alternatives could you try to help yourself right now? Be kind to yourself, not angry or critical. Just as it is when we are trying to understand the feelings of others, you will be amazed at how powerful a little understanding can be when it is extended toward yourself.

And last but not least, please don't forget to recognize your achievements. We are all brilliant at finding our flaws, but it can be much harder to acknowledge when we have done well. Don't be afraid of setting yourself mini-targets and planning non-food rewards if you think that might help. For some people, just the satisfaction of a fully ticked habit diary or Positive Nutrition Pyramid (see page 93) is reward enough. For other people, a shopping trip, spa treatment or other treat is the boost that they need to keep them driving forward. So how are you going to give yourself a pat on the back when you need it?

Chapter Three:
POSITIVE NUTRITION

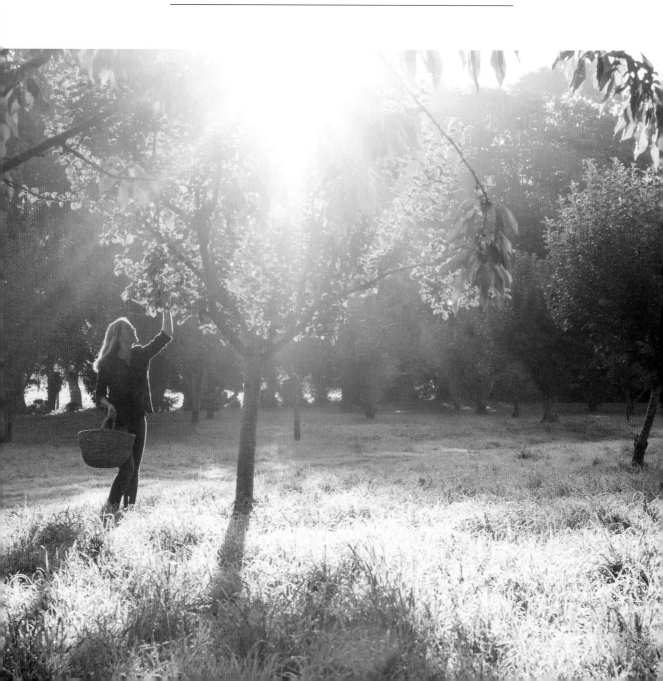

"Positive Nutrition is about eating better, not about eating less. It is about giving your body all of the fuel that it needs to function optimally, and is not about starving your body to fulfill perceived expectations."

I AM BEWILDERED AND SADDENED BY THE HUGE AMOUNT OF NEGATIVITY THAT NOW SURROUNDS SO MANY OF OUR FOOD CHOICES. There seems to be a constantly expanding list of foods that must be avoided, resisted, or only consumed as a "cheat," or "guilty pleasure." Foods have been labelled as either "clean" or "dirty"—a value judgment often based on nothing but marketing. Yet denying ourselves the joy of nourishing food is to deny ourselves one of the simplest pleasures in life. We have to eat, so it seems a huge shame that this essential part of our day can be so fraught.

I find myself working with an increasing number of clients who now feel intense fear around food. They have spent years removing its enjoyment, and instead have replaced pleasure with guilt and self-loathing.

And this is made harder by the so-called "rules" changing on an almost weekly basis. Something that was fine to include in our diet yesterday must supposedly be blacklisted today.

It is no wonder that some of us are feeling a tad disheartened and confused when it comes to food. If this resonates with you, then please rest assured—you are most certainly not alone.

"Lifestyle is about eating, not about dieting."

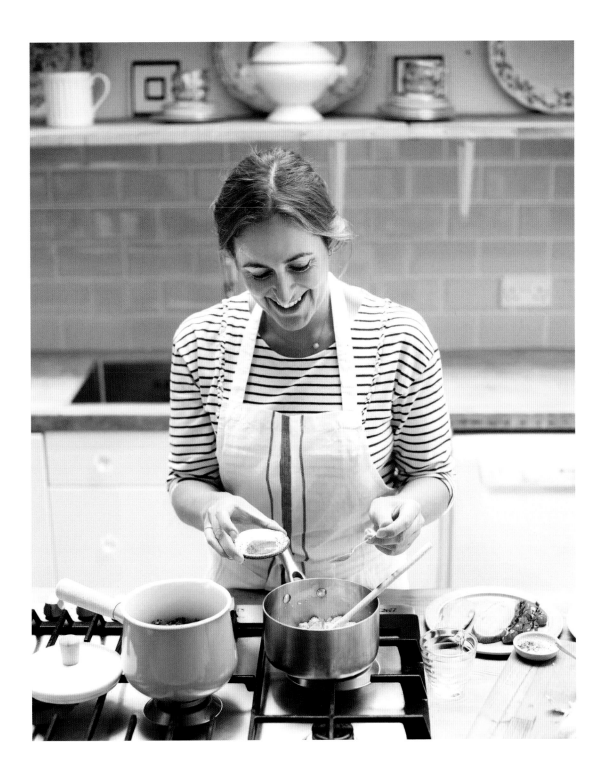

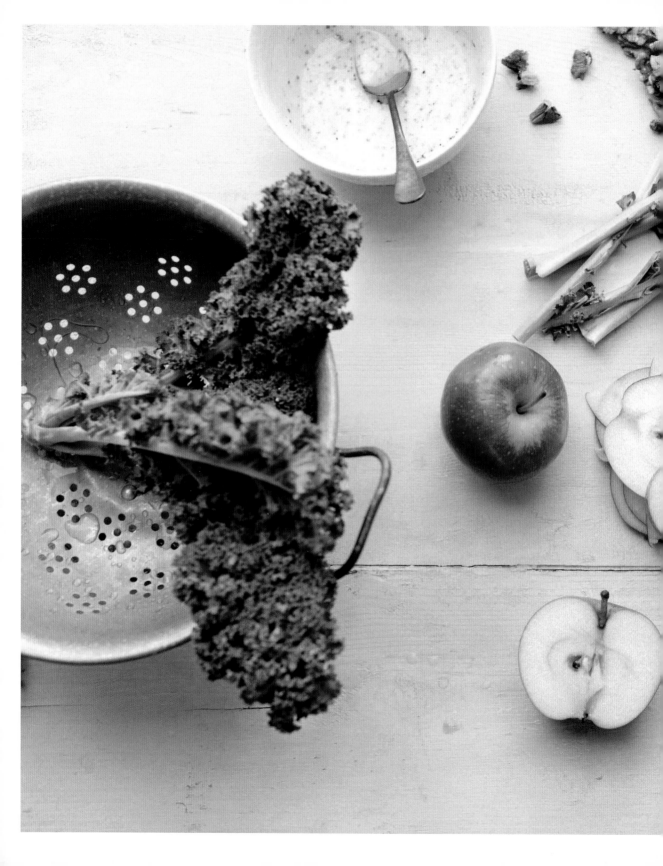

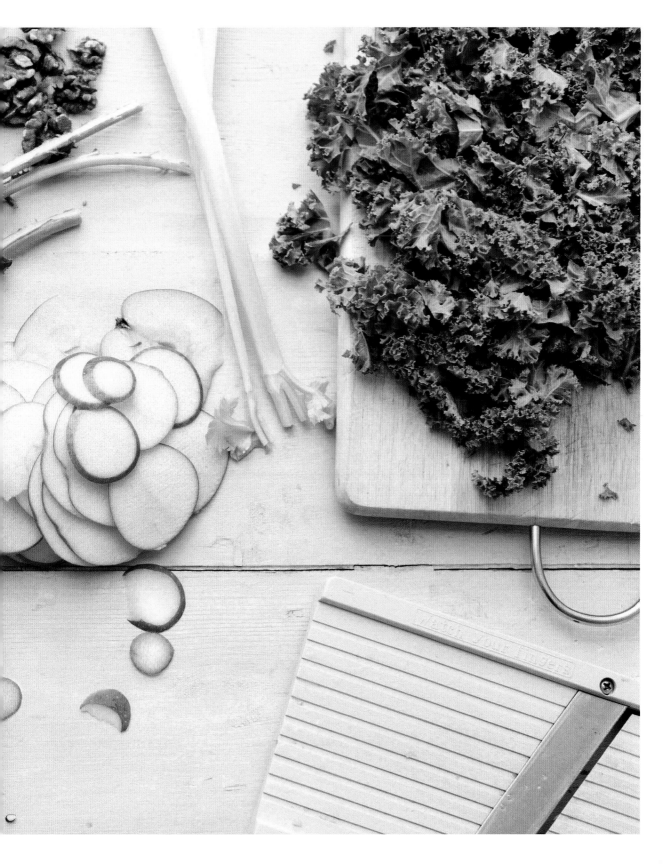

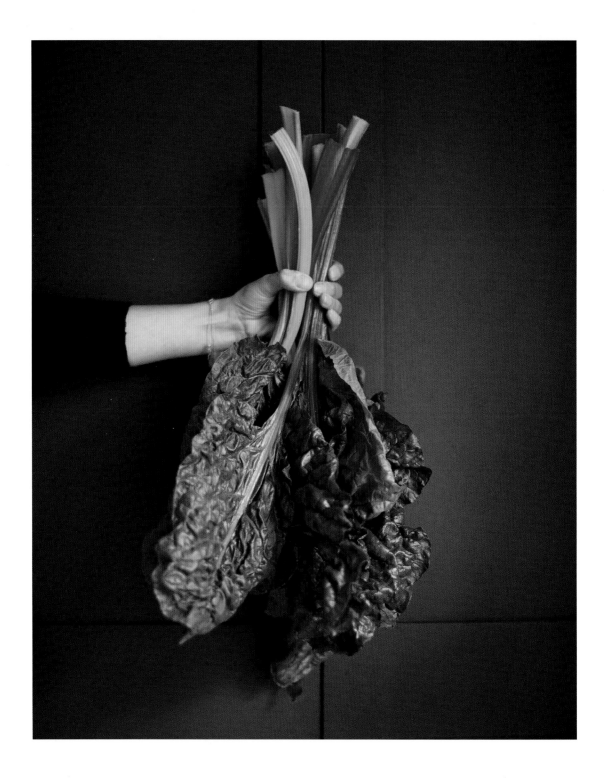

POSITIVE NUTRITION

I like to work in a positive mind-set and I always ask my clients to do this when we start working together. I begin by unpacking their set views on "dieting," and asking them to trust me, and together we wipe the slate clean. Now I am asking the same of you. Forget what's happened in the past. Forget the trends and marketing hype (however convincing it might seem). Forget the calorie-counting and the "clean" labels. But most of all, forget the worry, fear, or inhibition you may have around food. Instead, let's build things back up again together, from more positive, contented foundations.

I want to start by focusing not on what you *can't* have to eat, but on what you *can and should* have to eat. Every. Single. Day. This ensures your body has the chance to obtain all of the vital nutrition that it needs to function properly. Embracing this concept can help to disarm lots of those powerful thoughts of deprivation and fear surrounding food choices or diets. I therefore call it Positive Nutrition.

For our bodies to work in optimal condition we need to make sure that we are getting plenty of essential nutrients, while still maintaining a sensible energy balance. As well as the important "macronutrients"—like carbohydrates, fats, and proteins—there are *over* 40 "micronutrients" too (vitamins, minerals, essential fatty acids, and amino acids). Each of these has a key role in our body. Despite the various controversies in the world of science over what constitutes an "essential" nutrient, the key point is that there are a lot!

Vitamins:

- A (retinol)
- B1 (thiamine)
- B2 (riboflavin)
- B3 (niacin)
- B5 (pantothenic acid)
- B6 (pyroxidine)
- B7 (biotin)
- B9 (folate)
- B12 (cobalamin)
- C
- D
- E (tocopherol)
- K

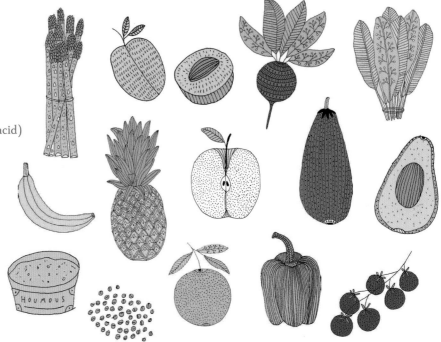

Essential amino acids:

Animal protein is "complete" protein because each serving contains all these amino acids. Some vegetable proteins, such as quinoa and spirulina, are also complete.

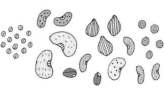

- Histidine
- Isoleucine
- Leucine
- Lysine
- Methionine
- Phenylalanine
- Threonine
- Tryptophan
- Valine

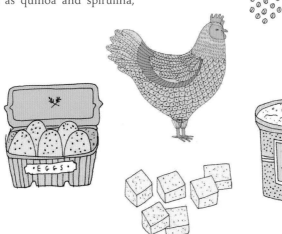

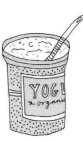

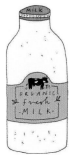

Minerals:

- Calcium
- Chromium
- Cobalt
- Copper
- Iodine
- Iron
- Magnesium
- Manganese
- Molybdenum
- Phosphorus
- Potassium
- Selenium
- Sodium
- Zinc

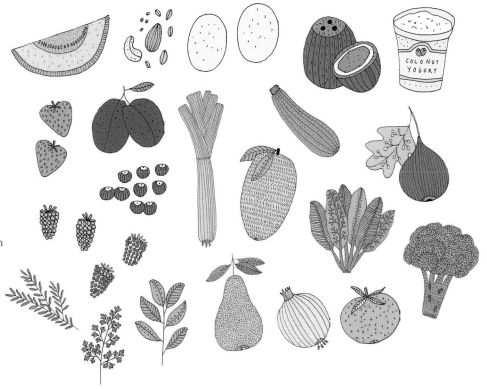

Essential fatty acids:

- Alpha-Linolenic Acid (omega-3)
- Linolenic Acid (omega-6)

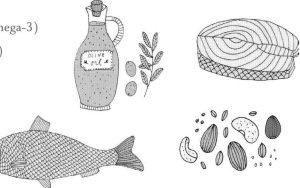

Positive Nutrition therefore begins with compassion toward ourselves, and an understanding that our bodies need to be fueled properly. Energy balance is still important, but calories are just one small part of nutrition; yet so often we seem to focus (sometimes obsessively) only on them.

It is important to point out that this book was not written specifically with weight loss in mind. Instead, it is designed to help you achieve your own version of a healthy, well-balanced, and varied diet *for life*, packed full of the nutrition you need to thrive. That is not to say that if you have some weight to lose, it won't help you to start losing it. However, this should be a steady and sustainable weight loss, not the dramatic short-term loss that is the result of many crash or fad diets. I find that when anyone begins to eat well, weight loss is usually a natural side effect. But calories and weight are definitely not the main focus here.

A healthy and sustainable diet is therefore one that is abundantly filled with all sorts of nourishing and delicious foods. Those foods should predominantly be *whole* foods.

I am often asked what "whole foods" really means, as it is a term that is often used but rarely defined.

- A whole food has just one ingredient—itself.
- It is very minimally processed, if at all, and is recognizable from its natural form.

WHOLE FOOD	NOT A WHOLE FOOD (more than one ingredient or processed)
Whole rolled oats	Instant oats or breakfast cereals
Navy beans	Canned baked beans
An orange	Orange juice
Plain hazelnuts	Hazelnut and chocolate spread
A roast chicken	Chicken nuggets
A fresh tomato	Jarred tomato pasta sauce

Whole foods are things like fresh fruit and vegetables, minimally processed grains, beans, and other legumes (like chickpeas or lentils), unprocessed meat, fish and shellfish, eggs, nuts, and seeds. Basing a diet predominantly on these ingredients means you will (hopefully!) never wander too far off the right nutritional path.

We don't have to just eat single ingredients though. We can combine whole foods into meals, and yes—I suppose that that does mean that we are processing them in some way. But the difference between home cooking and buying ready-processed food can be huge.

Commercial refining, processing, shaping, and packaging may result in foods with increased *energy* density (the amount of calories your body absorbs during digestion) while simultaneously decreasing the *nutrient* density (the concentration of vitamins, minerals, fiber, and so on) compared to the original ingredients. And that doesn't even take into account any artificial additives that might be included along the way.

Perhaps one of the best things about eating a mainly whole-foods diet is that we actually don't need to worry so much about energy balance or calories any more. As many whole foods are relatively low in energy density, or are highly satisfying and filling, it becomes harder to accidentally overeat. And even if we do end up eating a little too much, we will still be getting lots of healthy benefits alongside that energy. But as I mentioned in Chapter One, we are far less likely to feel the need to overeat if we do not feel like we are restraining ourselves around food in the first place. Letting go of the reins and embracing abundant whole food nutrition promotes a virtuous cycle: the less you're constantly holding yourself back around food, the less you're likely to need to. And let's not ignore the addictive qualities of many junk foods, which can trap so many of us into negative cycles of cravings, constant hunger, and decreased energy.

Thankfully, much of this is also common sense. A huge plate of salad, steamed vegetables, legumes, and seeds fills our stomachs and our daily nutrient needs, but the same amount of energy consumed in a cake does neither. The more nutrient goodness we can pack into our daily energy requirements, the better.

That is not to say that we cannot enjoy frivolities and festivities on top of those healthy foundations, but Positive Nutrition is far less about saying "No" to less-healthy foods than it is about saying a great big "YES! YES! YES!" to all of the gloriously nourishing whole foods instead.

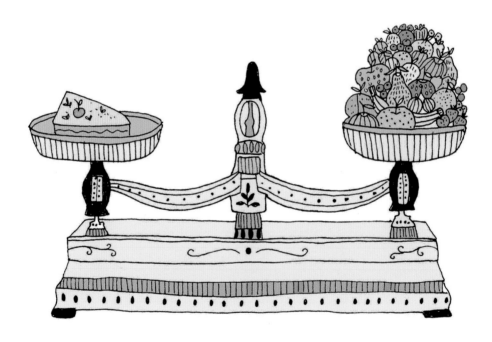

ENERGY SCALES

Positive Nutrition

THE HEALTHY RIPPLE EFFECT

Case study: Beyond Weight Loss

Mrs. X was in her fifties. After a lifetime in a stressful and demanding career, raising children and looking after the household, she had found herself gradually putting on weight. By the time I saw her, Mrs. X's self-esteem was at rock bottom and she told me she felt "disgusting" in her own skin. A health scare had prompted her to get some nutritional help.

We worked together to start undoing her detrimental eating habits, and gradually Mrs. X started to reduce her reliance on fatty, sugary comfort foods, choosing more fresh, nourishing whole foods instead. As the weight started to drop off, she began to feel confident again. She lost forty pounds and ten years off her appearance.

But it was the positive ripple effect that was perhaps most impressive to witness. As Mrs. X's self-esteem had plummeted, her emotional reliance on others had become almost suffocating. This, understandably, was starting to threaten her relationships. Yet with her transformation came a blossoming of her self-esteem. She no longer felt "disgusting." She tried on new clothes and felt beautiful again. People paid her compliments (and rightly so—she was positively glowing), and she started to invest more time and effort in herself. And with this improved self-belief, she also began to relax more, to let go of those she had needed to cling so tightly to for support. She felt able to change her job, spend more time with her friends, and the relationship she had with her husband was transformed back into what it had been when they first met.

The effects of Mrs. X's nutritional changes went so far beyond just food: not only was she fundamentally healthier and happier, but those around her felt more contented too. This was a wonderful example of the "healthy ripple effect."

It is very difficult to predict ahead of time how far your own ripple effect will go once you embark on new healthy habits, but it's safe to say that it will go somewhere. Even if you start off by making positive changes just for yourself, you may well find that you end up helping others along the way too, and that in itself can be a great motivating factor.

Try to remember that what you are doing is definitely not just a diet—this is about life, about health, about relationships, and about your own happiness. It might seem like those are bold claims to make, but I have seen this first hand so often that I genuinely believe it to be true. And isn't that a more cheerful thought to start from, than one that critically says "just eat less and move more"?

As I mentioned above, weight loss may well be a beneficial side effect if you have weight to lose, but as a concept, Positive Nutrition can offer you so much more than that. So I urge that your focus should now be on working toward establishing and becoming comfortable with your own interpretation of Positive Nutrition, and *not* about weight—you'll likely find that doing this takes an awful lot of pressure off too.

BUILDING BLOCKS OF A HEALTHY DIET:
thinking about time frames

Now we have explored the fundamental principles of Positive Nutrition, we can move on to how to put it into practice. First is an important explanation of one of the key ways I think about my own nutrition.

I tend to divide what I eat into four time frames, which, on reflection, is what helps me to plan and maintain a nutritionally balanced diet over the long term. Remember, consistency is key here. Expecting perfection in every time frame will inevitably be impossible to maintain.

1. Individual meals

This is where I tend to be quite flexible. After all, we cannot always predict what will happen during the course of a day, and some meals will not always turn out quite as planned. So don't beat yourself up over a single meal that isn't as healthy as you'd like it to be. It is what you do repeatedly that makes an impact, not what you do occasionally.

In general, I try to get at least some protein, healthy fats, and either fruit or vegetables at every meal. The forms of these nutrients vary hugely, and are usually chosen on a whim, depending on how I'm feeling and what's in the kitchen or on offer.

2. The whole day

Over the course of a whole day, at least when I am able to, I like to make sure that I have got at least my basic foundations covered—things like getting enough protein, fresh fruit and vegetables, water, healthy fats, etc. So that means that if one meal was a little weak, nutritionally speaking, I will make a bit of an effort to boost my other meals that day.

There are infinite variations in how I achieve the balance I am after, so I never feel constrained. I have developed a tool called the Positive Nutrition Pyramid (see the following page) to help me achieve this, which I find extremely helpful (and hopefully you will too!)—but we will explore this in more detail a little later on.

3. A week

There are a couple of things I aim for which don't need to be thought about as often as once a day. Handily, I call this my "rule of twos": I like to make sure that I am getting two portions of fish and, ideally, no more than two portions each of red meats and smoked/processed meats or fish per week. Simple!

4. A year

Overall health, energy levels, digestive function, skin, hair, nails, and mood are some of the best feedback mechanisms there are to let us know if our dietary changes are working or not, and these things take a little while to adapt. Plus, I am a great believer in eating with the seasons, not only because the food is often higher in nutrients (less farm-to-fork time means it is fresher when it reaches our kitchens), but because it is often tastier and more ecologically friendly, and it brings more variety to my plate.

I find using these time frames to be a really useful trick. It reminds me to not worry too much about the little details of every meal, but also helps guide me to stay on track in the longer term. I hope it helps you too.

THE POSITIVE NUTRITION PYRAMID

The dietary principles of Positive Nutrition are based on an adapted version of the Mediterranean diet.

Traditionally eaten by people who live close to the Mediterranean Sea in Italy, France, Greece, and Spain, it is a diet based on fruits and vegetables, lean sources of both plant and animal proteins, healthy fats from seeds, nuts, and oily fish, as well as generous amounts of olive oil. It is a well-researched diet and has been associated with a whole host of health benefits. Positive Nutrition also promotes these healthy foods, but our principles do diverge slightly when it comes to consuming lots of grains and daily wine (sorry!).

The Positive Nutrition Pyramid is a simple collection of circles, each of which represents a single portion of whole foods (such as "fresh fruit" or "nuts and seeds"). The aim of the game is to tick every circle by consuming all of the portions that one pyramid suggests every day. Each circle represents one portion of that food group. The whole pyramid represents one day of eating.

The Positive Nutrition Pyramid

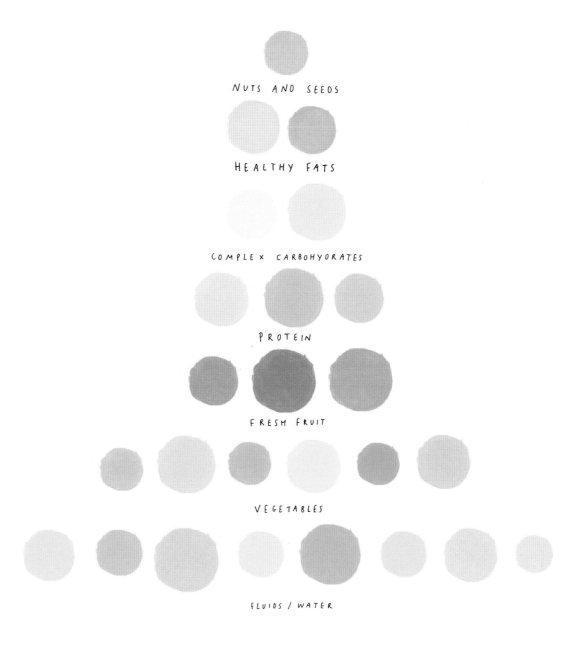

NUTS AND SEEDS

HEALTHY FATS

COMPLEX CARBOHYDRATES

PROTEIN

FRESH FRUIT

VEGETABLES

FLUIDS / WATER

With a little practice, the pyramid will start to help you to plan your meals and choose healthier options. After you have had breakfast and lunch, for example, you can then see exactly which circles still need to be ticked for your evening meal. You can then prepare a meal that incorporates those portions to complete the pyramid for the day. If you're a little confused at this point, don't worry, it will become more clear.

Most importantly the pyramid doesn't specify or restrict what you choose to eat *on top* of the portions recommended. The circles do not represent a maximum; they represent a suggested minimum. In fact, you'll find that the 10-day meal plan often goes above and beyond the various recommended portions each day.

That doesn't mean that I am encouraging a completely free rein to eat whatever you want, whenever you want. The pyramid will *only* work when it is your first priority in terms of your food budget, cooking and eating time, and, most importantly, your appetite. It is then up to you if you wish to add in foods or drinks that may be nice, but not necessary.

You will have gathered by now that this whole book is far more about what you should be eating, what you *need* to be eating, than what you shouldn't be eating or what is "banned." If there is nothing you are being asked to deprive yourself of, then there is nothing to feel deprived about! The joy of using Positive Nutrition is that by filling yourself up with naturally nutritious whole foods, over time you'll often find yourself wanting a smaller amount (if any) of those less healthy foods anyway.

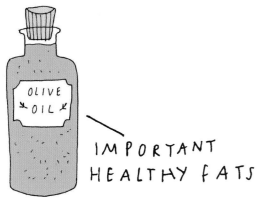

OLIVE OIL

IMPORTANT HEALTHY FATS

PROTEIN- PLUS SOME HEALTHY FISH OILS

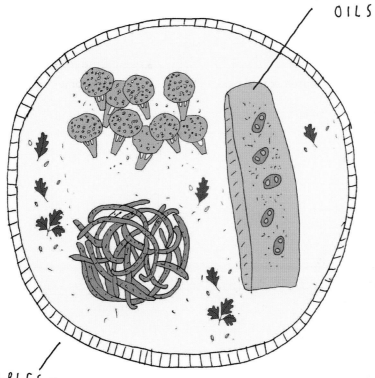

VEGETABLES- FOR LOTS OF VITAMINS, MINERALS, FIBER, AND EVEN SOME CARBOHYDRATES

FRESH FRUIT- FOR EVEN MORE VITAMINS, FIBRE AND PHYTONUTRIENTS

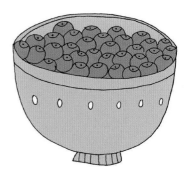

PUTTING THE POSITIVE NUTRITION PYRAMID INTO PRACTICE

Putting this all into practice is definitely *not* an exact science. There is no such thing as the perfect diet, but I think that this is a pretty good place for you to start from.

The basic principles

By the end of each day, you should have consumed all of the portions suggested in the pyramid. So that means six portions of veggies, three portions of fruit, etc. I did say this isn't about starvation! If you don't manage it all to start with, do not worry. I definitely don't want you to be trying to stuff yourself with any remaining portions or glugging five glasses of water just before bedtime. Try to spread the portions out across all three meals, and if you don't manage every circle by bedtime, don't worry about it.

- Start with just one thing. Choose one of the food groups that you know you often don't eat enough of (say, nuts and seeds), and incorporate that into your normal daily meals for a week, before adding another circle (say, a fruit one), and so on until you have built up to the whole pyramid. There is no shame in doing this slowly rather than going all-in at once. If it feels overwhelming, try drawing your own modified pyramid to start with.

- Don't worry about trying to "catch up" the following day if you miss a few portions. Each morning, just start afresh and have a try.

- As is often the case with nutrition, not all food categories are simple and straightforward. For example, a handful of almonds can be either "nuts and seeds" or "protein" or "healthy fats." Half a can of chickpeas could be either "starchy carbohydrates" or "protein." But one portion of food cannot count as all of these. One portion of food = one circle on the pyramid. It is therefore up to you to choose whichever circle you most need. Don't get too worried or caught up by this uncertainty. The reason I suggest you don't use one portion of food to tick off lots of circles is that I really want you to get as *wide* a variety of foods into your diet as possible to optimize your nutrient intake.

- Try to make the pyramid your first priority. If you find yourself eating foods or having drinks that do not fall under any of the circles on the pyramid, of course that is fine. But just to be clear, a cake cannot be a "starchy carbohydrate" nor a blueberry muffin a "fruit" portion!

- The pyramid that I have created is just a starting point. Tweak the circles or portions to suit your own appetite and requirements. In fact, I would be over the moon if you did so, because it shows that you are tuning in to your body and adapting your diet to suit your needs.

I never got along with very technical, precise nutritional programs, where I had to count calories, weigh food, or scan in barcodes to tell me how much I should be eating. I have always been a much more intuitive sort of judge. If it looked about right and felt about right, I would go for it. But I completely understand that this approach might be confusing for lots of people. The Positive Nutrition Pyramid portion guides therefore sit somewhere in between. They are *rough* outlines of what I would consider to be a portion, just to get you started, but are most certainly open to interpretation.

This is exactly how I want it to be, though. As I have said many times already, your body is utterly unique. What you need in a day will be different from what others need. And those needs will also change over time. A "good" diet is therefore a fluid and flexible thing. And if you pay enough attention, eat mindfully, and choose sensibly, your body will be the best guide that there is. Although the principles of a healthy diet may be common to most of us, their nuances, details, and interpretation are as varied as we are.

There can also be enormous variations between the foods themselves. An apple could be tiny or huge, depending on the variety. A chicken breast the same. There need be no anxiety or stress trying to aim for some sort of impossible "perfection" with the Positive Nutrition Pyramid. Please use your common sense and don't worry if you are making a best guess. It is, after all, only food—and therefore nothing to be scared of.

This picture shows you what a typical Positive Nutrition Pyramid might look like in real life: lots of beautiful, colorful portions of whole foods, covering all the important food groups.

But when I look at this picture, I also see an abundance of ingredients, and countless possibilities for how to combine them into tasty meals. Think of a variety of nutritious foods, such as these, as being your nutrition "toolkit." With the right tools for the job, and a little instruction (which you are holding in your hands right now!), you are in an excellent position to make healthy eating a real pleasure, and definitely not a chore.

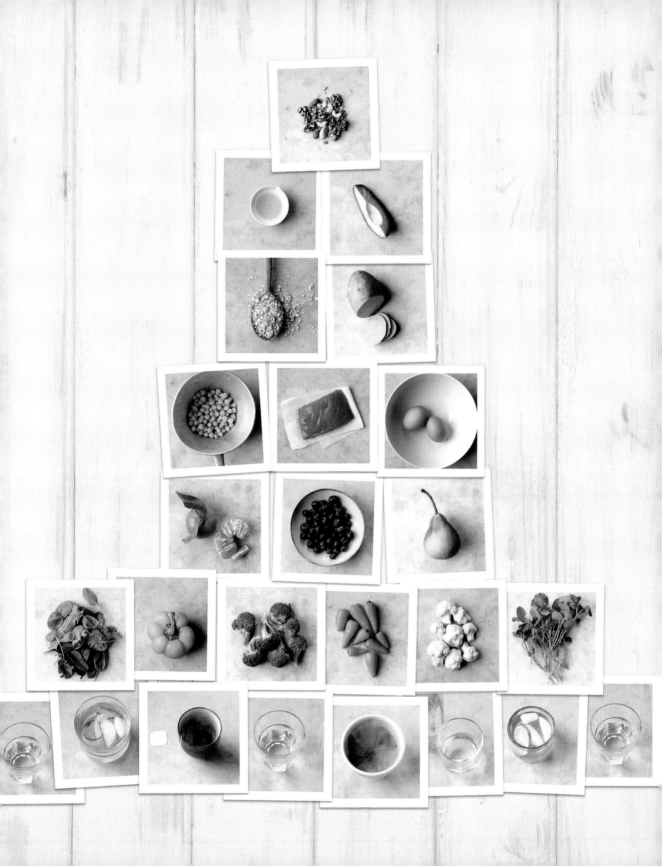

"Although the principles of a healthy diet may be common to most of us, their nuances, details, and interpretation are as varied as we are."

Protein: 3 portions per day
(a portion is approximately the size of your palm)

Protein is critical for growth and repair of tissues, as well as stabilizing our blood sugars and helping us to feel full. Three portions a day allows for one at breakfast, lunch, and dinner. You may find that you need slightly smaller or larger sized portions depending on your appetite, but I recommend that you try to get at least *some* protein into each of your meals.

Protein doesn't mean just meat or fish; you could use eggs or any number of plant-based proteins too (such as legumes, beans, nuts, or seeds).

THINGS TO BE CONSCIOUS OF:

- Try to avoid consuming processed or smoked meats (such as ham, cured meats, bacon, and sausages) too regularly.

- Mix up your sources—don't rely too heavily on one particular source of protein above another as they each have their own benefits. Personally, I don't like the taste of protein powders and so I focus more on whole-food sources.

- For ecological, animal welfare, and health reasons, I generally don't eat red meat more than twice a week, and I always try to buy it locally and organically.

- Try to eat fish 2–3 times a week. One of those portions should be an oily fish such as salmon, trout, mackerel, herring, or sardines, for its beneficial omega-3 fats. Look for wild, sustainably caught varieties wherever possible. Often cost-effective wild fish fillets can be found in the freezer section of the supermarket.

- I usually get at least one of my portions of protein from plants every day (such as some almonds at breakfast or hummus at lunch). This is good for the environment and my bank balance too!

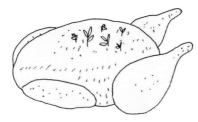

Around 4–5 oz lean (cooked)
meat—chicken, beef, turkey, game, etc.

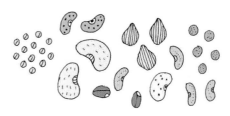

4 tablespoons cooked pulses—
chickpeas, lentils, or beans, etc.

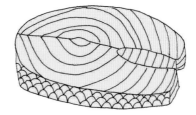

1 average fillet of fish

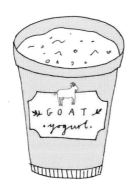

½ cup organic, plain yogurt
(I prefer sheep's or goat's milk yogurt
to cow's milk personally)

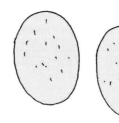

2 medium eggs
(ideally organic or
free-range)

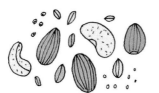

A small handful of nuts
or seeds (around 1 oz),
unsalted

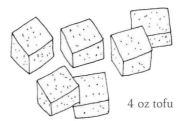

4 oz tofu

Complex carbohydrates: 2 portions per day
(a portion is approximately one cupped handful)

We get plenty of carbohydrates from fruit and vegetables, as well as from plant-based proteins such as beans and peas. I have therefore suggested that these carbohydrate portions can be optional. Minimally processed whole grains and starchy carbohydrates contain their own beneficial nutrients though, so by all means include them should you feel you need to. Personally, I don't eat many grains, but if I do want them, I eat the ones that suit me as and when I need.

A couple of portions a day tends to be about right for most people, but if you are trying to lose weight, or are not very active, then you may need less. If you are very active, however, you might need a little more.

THINGS TO BE CONSCIOUS OF:

- Opt for the lowest-sugar, highest-fiber, and least processed carbohydrates you can find wherever possible. The more it looks like it did when it was growing, the better! This maximizes nutritional value while minimizing impact on blood sugars.

- If possible, look out for organic grains, as they are likely to have a lower pesticide residue than non-organic varieties. We are currently unsure what the effects on our health may be of eating even small amounts of these residues over a long period of time. If you are buying non-organic grains, always wash them well under running water before cooking.

- Variety is the key. It is quite easy to end up just eating the same old carbs week after week, but this limits the tastes and flavors in your food, and also limits your body's access to a wide variety of nutrients, so try to shake up your shopping list where you can.

Please note that gluten- or wheat-containing grains are not included in the 10-day meal plan.

EXAMPLES MIGHT INCLUDE:

- 3–4 sugar-free oatcakes
- 2–3 small potatoes (each about the size of an egg)
- 1 small sweet potato or baked potato

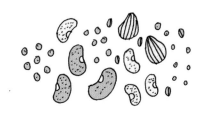

4 tablespoons of cooked pulses (such as beans, broad beans, lentils, legumes)

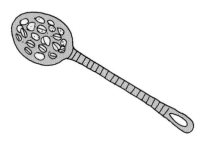

4–5 tablespoons of raw whole rolled oats

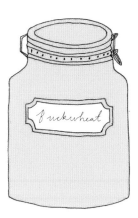
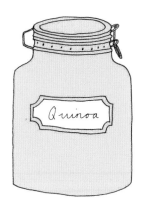
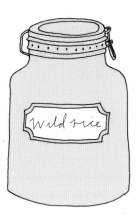

3–4 heaped tablespoons of cooked, unprocessed grains/seeds (such as brown or wild rice, quinoa, amaranth, buckwheat, barley, or millet)

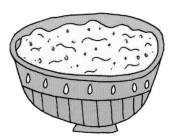

2–3 tablespoons of mashed potatoes, pumpkin, or squash

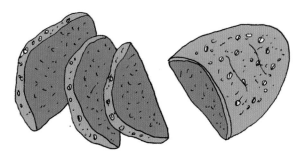

1–2 slices of bread—look out for rye, whole grain, buckwheat, or sourdough wherever possible

Healthy

(approxi

Dietary fa... ... the normal and health... ...energy-dense of all the f... ...n we want a few reason... ...r bodies the nutrients t... ...e scales too dramaticall...

EXAMPLES

- ¼ of a medium avocado
- 1 tablespoon of cooking or dressing oil (such as olive oil, avocado oil, or coconut oil)
- 1 tablespoon of nut butter or tahini
- 2 tablespoons of coconut yogurt
- ¼ can of full-fat coconut milk
- 1 oz (a small matchbox size) of cheese (I prefer sheep's or goat's milk cheeses, like chèvre or feta personally)
- A small handful of nuts or seeds (around 1 oz), unsalted

Please note: dairy fats are not included in the 10-day meal plan.

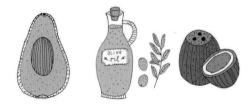

There is a difference between fats in terms of their potential health benefits, so I use a "traffic light" system when explaining this to clients:

RED

RED, AVOID:
Processed trans fats and hydrogenated fats (found most commonly in processed foods, margarine, pastry, cakes, and cookies), commercial salad dressings, oils heated repeatedly to high temperatures (such as those in deep-fat fryers), refined oils, such as sunflower oil, soybean oil, or "vegetable" oils.

AMBER

AMBER, EAT MINDFULLY:
Animal fats (such as those found in meat and dairy products).

GREEN

GREEN, EAT HAPPILY:
Oily fish (or fish-oil supplements), nuts, seeds, avocado, olive oil, and coconut fats.

TIP: If you have high cholesterol or a history of heart disease, I would generally advise sticking to olive oil as your cooking fat of choice. We know more about the benefits of olive oil in these circumstances at present.

Nuts and seeds: 1 portion per day
(a portion is approximately a small handful)

Nuts and seeds are wonderfully nutrient-dense foods, with a complex mixture of unsaturated fats, high-quality plant protein, minerals, fiber, and phytonutrients. Regular nut consumption has been linked to a reduced risk of coronary heart disease, high blood pressure, and cancer, and they may even support weight loss and help to lower cholesterol when enjoyed within a healthy diet.

I have therefore given nuts and seeds their very own box, because this encourages us to eat at least one portion per day. You may eat more than one portion though, as nuts and seeds can also be counted as a "healthy fat" or a "protein" circle too. But remember, one portion of food = just one circle on the pyramid. Stick to a maximum of about 3 oz (= 3 portions) per day.

EXAMPLES MIGHT INCLUDE:

- A small handful of nuts or seeds (around 1 oz), unsalted
- 1 tablespoon of nut butter or tahini

Nuts: Almonds, cashews, peanuts, pecans, walnuts, pistachios, macadamia nuts, pine nuts, Brazil nuts, hazelnuts, chestnuts

Seeds: Pumpkin, chia, sunflower, flaxseed, hemp, poppy, sesame

THINGS TO BE CONSCIOUS OF:

- Try to buy nuts and seeds as close to raw, whole, and unprocessed as possible. If you struggle to digest them, soak them in water in the fridge overnight.
- Try to eat a variety of nuts and seeds. Mixing it up makes sure you're

topping up your intake of all sorts of different nutrients, without going overboard on any in particular. Eating just one nut or seed in excess may increase the chance of developing a sensitivity further down the line too. I have seen this quite a lot with almonds since almond milk became so widely available. Another example would be Brazil nuts, which are one of our best sources of the essential mineral selenium, but you can eat too many; just 3–4 Brazil nuts a week is probably about right.

- Seeds can provide us with some omega-3 oils, but our bodies are not very efficient at converting the plant-based omega-3s into the important longer-chain omega-3s found in oily fish and fish-oil supplements. It's therefore best not to rely purely on nuts and seeds as your only source of omega-3 oils.

Fruit: 3 portions per day
(a portion is approximately the size of your clenched fist)

We have all heard the "five-a-day" motto, but in fact this is not the optimal number of fruit and vegetable portions for health. Ideally, we should be aiming for around *nine* portions of fruit and vegetables a day, and most of these should be vegetables, not fruit. I therefore encourage three portions of fruit—specifically fresh, whole fruit—per day for their beneficial nutrients but without too much fruit sugar.

If you are eating nowhere near this amount of fruit and vegetables at the moment (and don't worry if this is the case—the huge majority of the population is in the same boat), I suggest you don't try to go the whole hog all at once. It might feel a bit overwhelming to prepare. And all that extra fiber could cause some uncomfortable digestive symptoms. Instead, try increasing your intake by just one extra portion per day for a week or so to start with, gradually working your way up to more. If you are planning on doing the 10-day meal plan at the end of this book, then you might like to give yourself a couple of weeks of run-up time to do this before you start the program.

- 1 handful of large fruit chunks (such as mango, pineapple, melon)

- 1 medium-sized fruit (orange, pear, banana, apple, peach, nectarine, etc.)

- 2 pieces of small fruit (satsuma, clementine, plum, apricot, etc.)

- 2 large handfuls of berries (blueberries, blackberries, raspberries, strawberries, etc.)

- 1 handful of grapes—aim for black or red varieties for an antioxidant boost

- 2 heaped tablespoons of fruit compote/fruit puree

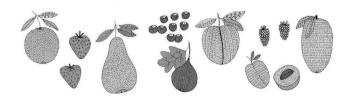

THINGS TO BE CONSCIOUS OF:

- If you cannot buy organic fruit, or if it is not a peelable variety, wash it thoroughly before eating.

- Don't rely on dried fruit. A couple of portions a week is fine, but they are higher in sugar and not as filling as whole fruits. The same goes for smoothies. It's fine to whizz up one portion of fruit (ideally alongside some veggies and a source of protein) into a smoothie occasionally, but it's better overall to try to eat most of your fruit whole.

- I do not count fruit juices as a portion of fruit—the fiber has been removed and they can be unhealthily high in sugar; one glass of orange juice can have as much sugar as a glass of soda.

- Try to eat the skins where they are edible as they provide fiber as well as beneficial antioxidants.

- Most of us have access to a true rainbow of colorful fruits to buy, so embrace it and eat vibrantly and with the seasons for maximum health benefits.

- Cooking fruit or vegetables at high temperatures and for long periods of time can destroy some heat-sensitive nutrients, so try to enjoy at least some of your fruit and vegetables raw. If you do need to cook them, steaming, baking, or quickly blanching are the best methods to minimize nutrient loss.

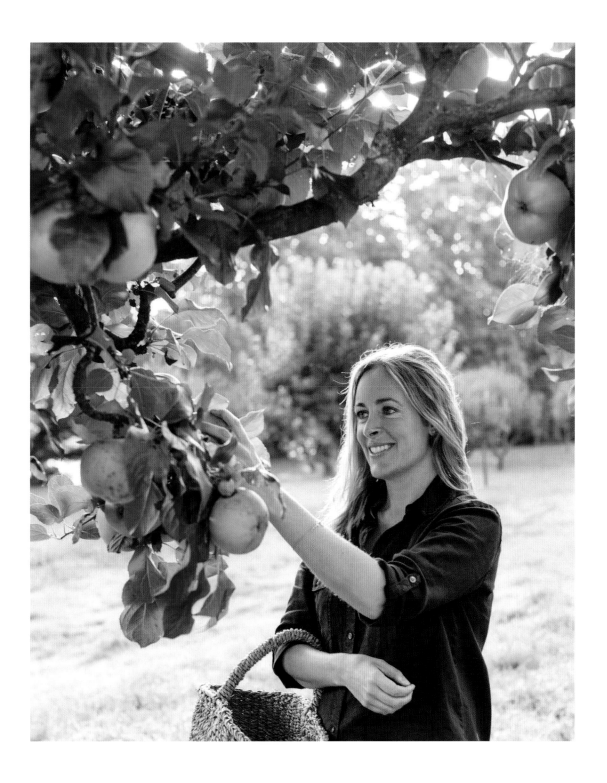

Vegetables: 6 per day
(a portion is approximately the size of your clenched fist; ideally 3 of these will be green vegetables)

Vegetables of all varieties are the basis on which a healthy diet is formed. Eating lots of them means that your meals will be filling and rich in vitamins, fiber, minerals, nutrients, and beneficial phytonutrients, without much energy density. I try to aim for around three of my six vegetable portions to be green (especially anything leafy—like kale, cabbage, spinach, fresh herbs, or salad leaves), although sometimes I eat a little more, and sometimes a little less. It depends on my mood, the seasons, and what I have available.

Don't be scared if this sounds like a lot of vegetables at first. As I keep saying, you don't have to do it all at once and can work up to this level slowly, maybe starting with just trying to get in one extra portion of vegetables a day.

EXAMPLES MIGHT INCLUDE:

- 1–2 handfuls of raw leafy greens (such as salad leaves, baby spinach, watercress, arugula, lamb's lettuce, baby Bibb lettuce leaves, etc.)
- 2–3 tablespoons of chopped fresh herbs
- 3 heaped tablespoons of chopped raw or cooked vegetables
- 1 carrot or stick of celery
- 1 medium zucchini, leek, or onion
- 2 medium tomatoes or a handful of cherry tomatoes
- ½ an eggplant or large pepper
- ¼–½ of a small head of cabbage

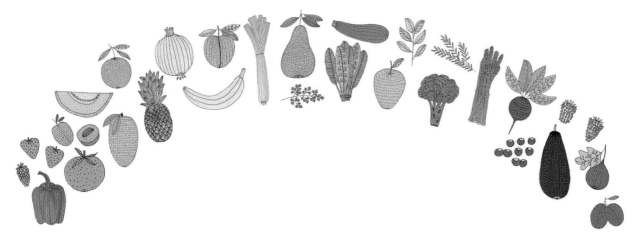

THINGS TO BE CONSCIOUS OF:

- Don't get too hung up on the exact sizes of your portions. Approximations and "guesstimates" are absolutely fine! You could make up one portion with half an onion and half a carrot, for example. Or tick two circles if you've had a particularly big helping of salad. You'll get the hang of it quickly by using the size of your clenched fist as your rough guide.

- Green leafy vegetables are a non-dairy source of calcium (which if you are vegan or reducing your dairy intake is good to know).

- Just as with fruit, try to eat a rainbow of colors in your vegetables, and when you can, eat with the seasons for maximum health benefits.

"It is far better to make easy changes that you are able to stick to for a lifetime than really hard changes that only last a week."

Fluids: approximately 8 medium glasses (68 oz) per day (although this may vary considerably depending on your personal needs)

It is actually a myth that we must drink 8 glasses of fluid a day (I didn't always know this!). But I have used it as a ballpark figure for what the average person might need to drink on the average day. It is also common to accidentally mistake thirst for hunger and end up unwittingly overeating trying to quench it. You may also need to up your fluid intake if you are increasing your fiber intake, to avoid digestive issues.

If it is really hot, or you're working or exercising hard, then you'll need more fluids. If you're fairly sedentary, you may need less. Pay attention to your own thirst as a guide, and you can keep an eye on your overall hydration status by drinking just enough fluid to keep your urine a very pale color.

EXAMPLES MIGHT INCLUDE:

- Plenty of water: water should make up the majority of your fluid intake in a day. If you don't like plain water, you could try adding slices of cucumber, lemon, orange, berries, or fresh herbs to a jug, bottle, or glass.

- Herbal teas

- Organic milk (personally, I like alternatives to dairy, such as almond or coconut milk. I tend to steer clear of soya milk, but if you do buy it, look out for an organic one.)

- Tea and coffee, in moderation (aim for no more than 1–2 cups of coffee or 3–4 cups of tea a day). If you are choosing a decaf version, look out for organic ones.

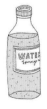

Positive Nutrition

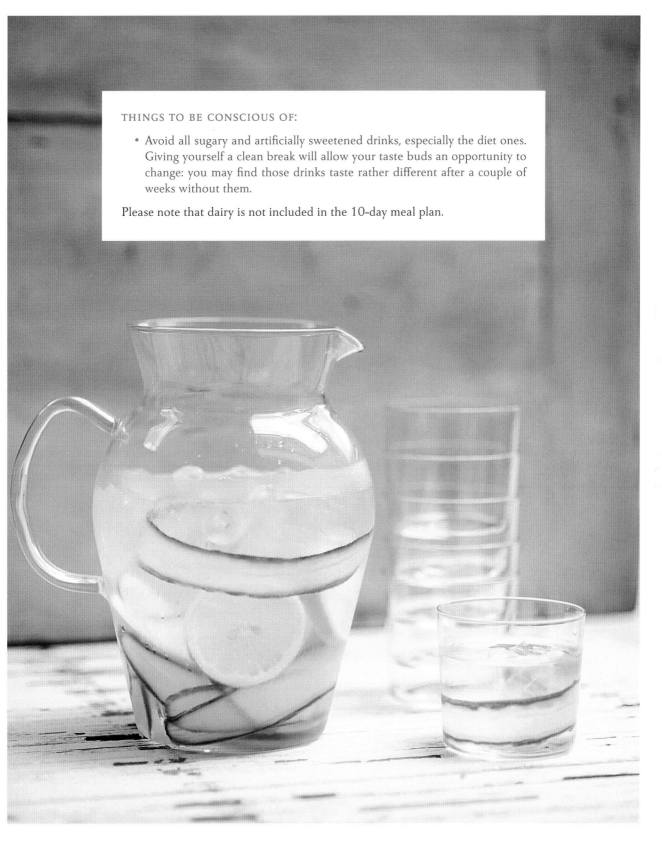

THINGS TO BE CONSCIOUS OF:

- Avoid all sugary and artificially sweetened drinks, especially the diet ones. Giving yourself a clean break will allow your taste buds an opportunity to change: you may find those drinks taste rather different after a couple of weeks without them.

Please note that dairy is not included in the 10-day meal plan.

CREATING THE OPTIMAL DIET FOR YOU

As I have said many times, although the broad principles of what makes up a healthy diet can be generalized for most people—things like eating minimal amounts of processed foods or refined sugars, and plenty of whole foods like fruits and vegetables—how they are fine-tuned varies enormously. A healthy, balanced diet for a sedentary woman in her eighties will look very different from that of a bodybuilder in his twenties. That is why one single "perfect" diet has never been found. It all depends on you.

So if the ideal diet for you is unique to your needs, what would you want your needs to be? Below are a few ideas; things that you may hope your own optimal diet will provide.

Is there anything else that you would add or take away from this list?

What do I want / need from my optimal diet?

- ✎ Pleasure and enjoyment—from both eating and preparing food
- ✎ Variety—of foods, of flavors, of seasonal produce
- ✎ All the essential micronutrients
- ✎ The right macronutrient balance for me: protein, carbohydrates, and fats
- ✎ Sustainability—it needs to fit into my lifestyle with ease
- ✎ To help me achieve a weight or body composition that is healthy for me
- ✎ The flexibility to enjoy my social life without anxiety or fear

And if you *were* enjoying your own optimal diet, how would you know that it was working well for your mind, body, and life? What sorts of symptoms would you expect? How would you feel? What might you be on the lookout for? These are the cues that your body can give you to let you know if you are on the right track, or if something might need a little adjustment.

Here are a few ideas. Are there any others that you would add to your list?

- I would be feeling full of energy and sleeping well at night.

- I'd be satisfied with each meal, rarely needing to snack between meals or finding myself craving certain foods.

- I would definitely be enjoying eating this way, and generally finding myself feeling full at the end of each meal.

- I would notice that I had strong nails, shiny hair, and glowing, clear skin. Other people might notice this too.

- My weight would be optimizing (sensibly increasing if I was underweight, gradually decreasing if was overweight, or staying steady if I was already a healthy weight).

- I would experience minimal digestive symptoms—bloating, gas, indigestion, stomach upsets, etc.

Chapter Four:
THE 10-DAY PLAN
TO NOURISH & GLOW

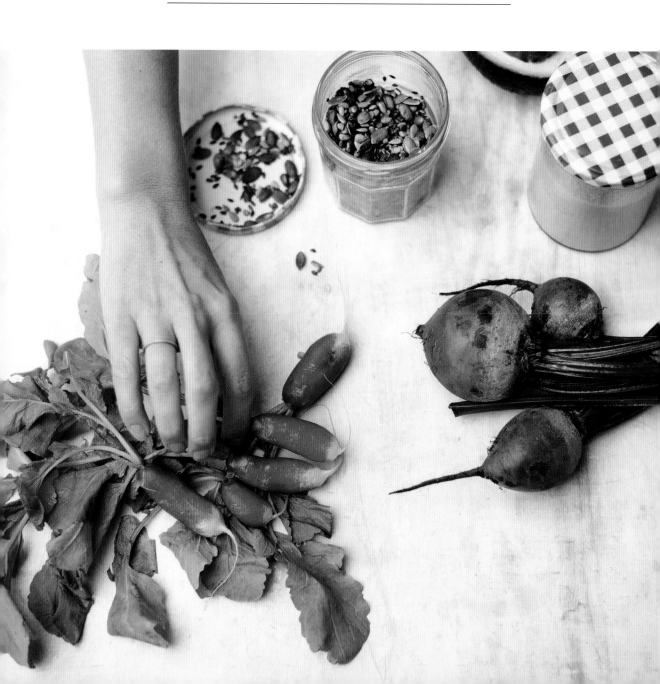

My main aim for you in this chapter is to learn what it really feels like to plan, shop, cook, and eat a nutritious, well-balanced, and varied diet for 10 days. The knowledge and insights that you can gain from putting this theory into practice within the context of your own busy life can be far more useful than reading it on a page.

If you are someone who loves to be given specific instructions, who relishes detailed guidance, and who likes to jump in feet-first, then this plan is definitely for you. My team and I have painstakingly planned and tested each day, ensuring that the Positive Nutrition Pyramid is fulfilled to maximize nutritional goodness. The simple but tasty recipes will help to ensure minimal food waste and use easily sourced ingredients as much as possible. I really hope that you enjoy the meals and the structure that the plan gives you.

However, if you are like me and sometimes struggle to follow a plan, then do not worry. Use it as a bit of guidance or inspiration, dipping in and out as you wish. Perhaps the plan could help to build up your

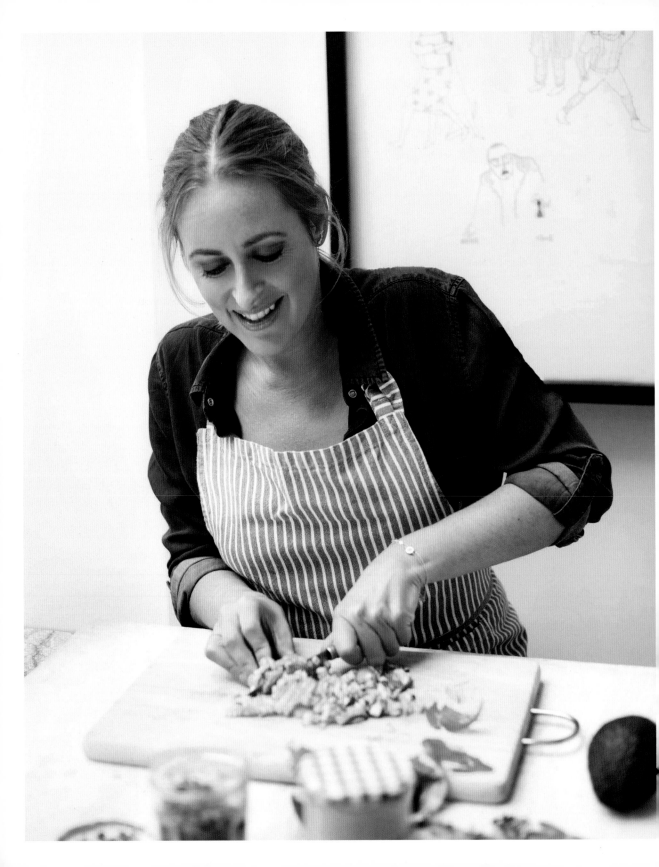

new habits, or it could help to support any step-by-step changes you decide to make. Meal plans work for some people, and don't for others. Just do what feels right for you.

Every day of the plan starts with a photograph of all the meals you will be having over the course of that day, in one place. I think that this visual guide is really useful as you can see what quantities of food and portion sizes are suggested, and also how beautiful, how colorful, how alive and vibrant it all looks. I hope you find this as inspiring as I do!

"When you recover or discover something that nourishes your soul and brings joy, care enough about yourself to make room for it in your life."
—Jean Shinoda Bolen

THE 10-DAY PLAN: HOW IT WORKS

I would encourage you to read through this section carefully before starting the 10-day plan as it should help you understand how it all works and give you some tips and tricks to get you started on the right track.

PLAN

- Have a look through the whole plan before making a start on it, so that you know what is involved and what sorts of things you'll be cooking and eating. Some of the recipes have alternatives and variations to try, or perhaps you'd prefer the vegan option for that day.

- If you are worried that the 10-day plan feels overwhelmingly different from how you normally eat, then ease yourself in a little more gently. Perhaps pick one layer of the pyramid—protein, for example—and start by just trying to make sure you are including a portion of protein with each of your usual meals for a couple of weeks. Then pick another part of the pyramid and do the same. This way, you can build up your confidence, before launching into the full program when you feel ready. There is no right or wrong way to approach this, so do what feels right for you.

- If you are a real caffeine addict, I suggest that you take a couple of weeks to wean yourself off it a little before starting the program. Dramatically reducing your caffeine intake can lead to headaches and fatigue. Perhaps try reducing by just a cup or two a day for a week (replacing them with herbal teas or water), aiming eventually to drink no more than 1–2 cups of coffee a day, or 3–4 cups of tea. Don't forget that chocolate and some fizzy drinks may contain caffeine too.

- If possible, try to choose a 10-day period in which to complete the plan that is relatively free of social commitments. We cannot live our lives avoiding social situations, but just for these first 10 days it's a good idea to avoid distractions or temptations.

SHOP

- Although there is a shopping list provided to accompany the meal plan (see pages 320–321), there will be regional and seasonal variations in what is available to you. There are very few (if any) recipes in this plan that could not take some degree of variation in the ingredients, so feel free to make alterations, substitutions, or swaps as you wish. You never know—you may even improve the recipe!

- Look out for local, free-range, and ideally organic meat if you can. The plan bulks out meals with lots of cheaper vegetables and pulses, so it is worth stretching your budget if possible. The same goes for eggs.

- It's a similar story for your fruit and vegetables. If you have a budget-friendly organic supplier, then fantastic. However, if you need to prioritize (and who doesn't), then I think the green leafy salads and soft fruit are the most important to buy organic. However, it's always better to eat a whole heap of non-organic fruit and vegetables than none at all.

- As soon as you have done the shopping for the plan, sort your groceries into a logical order in your kitchen cupboards and fridge. Being able to quickly lay your hands on the ingredients you are looking for saves a lot of time and hassle.

- When buying gluten-free bread, try to look for organic loaves. This is because all sorts of unusual ingredients can be used in the non-organic ones, trying to replicate the texture of "normal" bread. I tend to keep loaves in the freezer once opened and toasting the slices really well before eating. My favorites are either the millet or buckwheat varieties, but shop around to find the best for you. I know that gluten-free is not the cheapest option, but seeing as I only have maybe 2–3 slices a week, a small loaf will often last me a couple of weeks.

COOK

- Check that you have all the basic kitchen equipment that you will need for each day's cooking ready to go. A set of sharp knives, a great peeler, and an easily cleaned cutting board makes vegetable prep a less frustrating task.

- Have an old plastic bag or big mixing bowl next to you while preparing your vegetables. Any peelings, packaging, or offcuts go straight in there to help keep your workspace clean and clear.

- Throughout the meal plan, we will be using the "cook once, eat twice" idea to minimize the time spent cooking (and the dishwashing!). For food safety reasons, make sure that food is allowed to cool before putting it, covered, into the fridge or freezer. When you reheat something, make sure that it is piping hot before serving. Use your intuition: if something doesn't look, feel, or smell right to you, it is always better to leave it than risk giving yourself a nasty bout of food poisoning. No meal plan is worth that!

- Most recipes use either coconut or olive oil for cooking. Feel free to choose whichever you prefer. However, try to make sure that you avoid overheating or burning either oil—beyond the point at which both oils start "smoking," potentially harmful chemicals can form.

- All recipes serve one person, but sometimes make two portions if you are going to use the leftovers for another meal.

- Vegan alternative recipes are included with each day's recipes. When the main meal plan recipes are also vegan, you'll see a (v) next to the title. Check each day's menu for clarification. Some of the main meal plan recipes, that are also for the vegan plan, have a choice of sweetener in the ingredients list. If you are following the vegan plan, choose one of the options other than honey as honey is not a vegan product.

- At the end of each day of the plan you will find a "Complete Today's Preparation" section. This is designed to help you prepare for the next day after your evening meal: making breakfast or packed lunches if necessary, getting things out of the freezer, etc. Although just a guide, they might be particularly useful for the busy cook.

- In order to give you varied and original meals, I have devised lots of different recipes to include in this 10-day plan. I hope that they will give you plenty of new ideas, as well as increasing your cooking repertoire and skills. This may mean that you're spending a little more time cooking than normal. Rest assured, however, that day-to-day life doesn't need to be complicated. A bowl of steamed greens and a simple baked piece of fish is a delicious meal—but it doesn't necessarily make an exciting recipe! At the end of the plan, you can pick your favorites and mix them up and, hopefully, you'll find a way of eating that not only suits your taste buds but your time, budget, and overall health as well.

EAT

- The plan consists of three meals a day, no snacks. This might be hard to start with, especially if you are used to being a bit more of a "grazer," but I promise it does get easier. Make sure you are drinking plenty of water in between meals, and rest assured that it is perfectly natural and completely OK to feel a little hunger. So many of us have a real fear of it. The French have a lovely saying: "Hunger makes the best condiment"— and I really believe this to be true. Food just tastes better when you are a little hungry for it.

- I have made the meal plan gluten-, dairy-, and refined sugar-free. That is not to say that this is what I advise for everyone, but it allows you the opportunity to see whether you *feel* better without these ingredients, as many people do.

- While devising this meal plan, I have tried hard to ensure that each day you consume three portions of protein, three different pieces of fruit, a rainbow of colorful vegetables and healthy fats, which is heaps

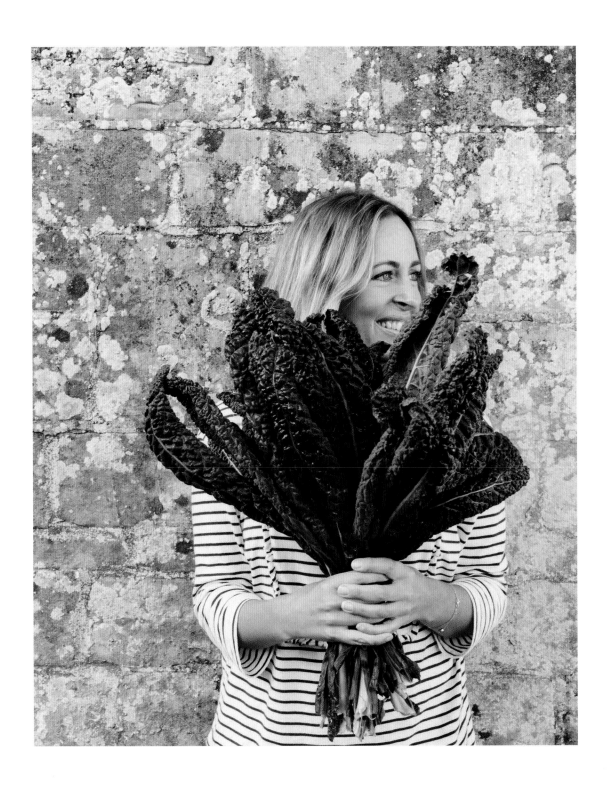

of nutrition, just as the Positive Nutrition Pyramid shows us. On some days there aren't a lot of starchy carbohydrates. This is because most people undertaking the 10-day plan would probably like to lose a bit of weight. If, however, you are very active or *not* trying to lose weight, then please add in some extra portions of starchy carbs to the days that don't include them. Perhaps add a portion of gluten-free toast to breakfast, a few gluten-free oatcakes to lunch, or a couple of potatoes to supper, for example. Likewise, if you are absolutely ravenous, you could always increase the size of the portions you are serving yourself slightly—or indeed if you are feeling very full, decrease their size. Listen to your body and honor what it is trying to say, and you won't go wrong.

- "Mindful moments" have been included, to emphasize the importance of eating slowly, sitting down, and taking time over your food. I often find with my clients that this step alone can make a huge difference.

- You might be wondering what to do about alcohol and "treats." I think it is best to stick as closely to the 10-day meal plan as possible to maximize the benefits you will feel and see. However, after the plan has finished, of course, there is always going to be space in your diet for special occasions. It's just a case of choosing the "worth it" moments.

At the beginning of each recipe is a key that corresponds to the Positive Nutrition Pyramid, so you can easily see which food groups the recipe contains. The number within each circle tells you how many portions there are of that food group, per serving.

| NUTS AND SEEDS | HEALTHY FATS | COMPLEX CARBOHYDRATES | PROTEIN | FRESH FRUIT | VEGETABLES | WATER OR FLUIDS |

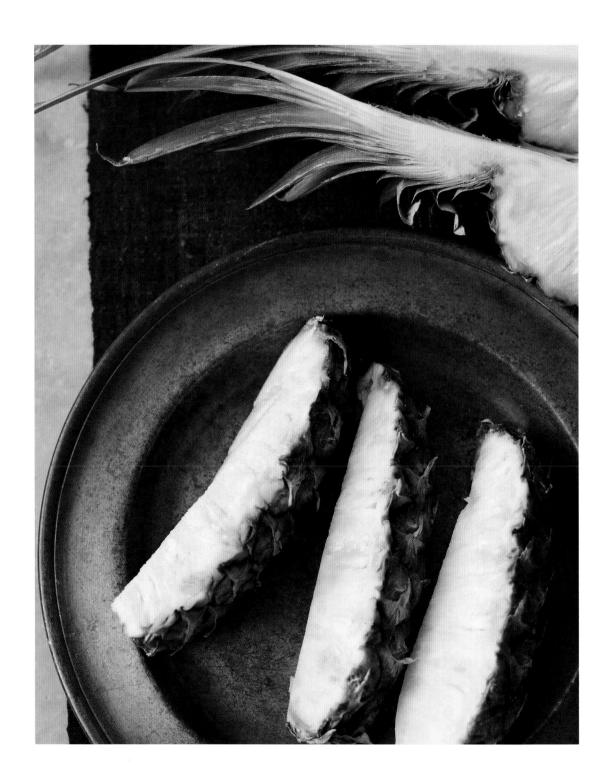

THE BACKUP PLAN

Sometimes unforeseen circumstances get in the way of even the best intentions. Meetings overrun, children get sick, cars break down . . . you get the idea. It's therefore always good to have a few very quick and simple meals up your sleeve, so you can stay on track whatever the day has thrown at you.

Here are some ideas to get you started. Preparing for these occasions means we're far less likely to fall off the wagon.

BREAKFAST	Nut granola with milk or a dollop of coconut yogurt + 1 portion of seasonal fruit
LUNCH	Simple fridge salad or store-brought vegetable soup, topped with ½ can of drained beans or chickpeas, a couple of tablespoons of toasted seeds, and a drizzle of extra-virgin olive oil + 1 portion of seasonal fruit
SUPPER	Some roughly chopped soft vegetables (zucchini, peppers, tomatoes, etc.), stir-fried with a couple of eggs to make a quick hash Serve on a slice of gluten-free toast and a handful of salad leaves

MENU

Prep day recipes:

Beet Hummus (page 136) (v)

Spiced Seed Sprinkle (page 140) (v)

Nut Granola (page 141) (v)

Day 1

Breakfast: Turmeric & Mango Spiced Chia Pot (page 148) (v)

Lunch: Rainbow Abundance Bowl + 1 portion of seasonal fruit (page 151) (v)

Supper: Roast Chicken with Roasted Vegetables (page 152) + 1 portion of seasonal fruit

Day 2

Breakfast: Breakfast Frittata (page 167) + 1 portion of seasonal fruit

Lunch: Chicken Pâté in lettuce cups (page 168) + 1 portion of seasonal fruit

Supper: Wild Salmon Parcels with Asian-style Salad (page 171) + 1 portion of seasonal fruit

Day 3

Breakfast: Banana, Mint & Lime Smoothie (page 182) (v)

Lunch: Salmon Salad in a Jar (page 185) + 1 portion of seasonal fruit

Supper: Eggplant & Chickpea Curry (page 186) (v) + 1 portion of seasonal fruit

Day 4

Breakfast: Overnight Oat Crumble with Apple (page 196) (v)

Lunch: Leftover Eggplant & Chickpea Curry (page 186) (v) + 1 portion of seasonal fruit

Supper: Grilled Fish with Orange & Avocado Salsa (page 198)

Day 5

Breakfast: Overnight Oat Crumble with Berries (page 196) (v)

Lunch: Roasted Vegetable & Chicken Soup (page 206) + 1 portion of seasonal fruit

Supper: Spicy Tomato & Shrimp Zucchini Noodles (page 209) + 1 portion of seasonal fruit

Day 6

Breakfast: Nut Granola with Berries
(page 219) (v)

Lunch: Smoked Salmon & Kale Waldorf Salad
(page 220)

Supper: Chicken & Chips with Chopped
Salad (page 222) (v) + Nutty Banana Nice
Cream (page 227)

Day 7

Breakfast: Pea & Sweet Potato Fritter
(page 239) + 1 portion of seasonal fruit

Lunch: Chopped Chicken Salad (page 240)

Supper: Fish Goujons with Tartar Sauce
(page 242) + Nutty Chocolate Pot (page 245) (v)

Day 8

Breakfast: Herby Green Omelet (page 259)
+ 1 portion of seasonal fruit

Lunch: Smoked Salmon Pâté with
vegetable crudités and oatcakes (page 260) (v)
+ 1 portion of seasonal fruit

Supper: Stuffed Peppers with Chili (page 262) (v)
+ Baked Orange & Almond Pear (page 266) (v)

Day 9

Breakfast: Baked Pear Breakfast Bowl
(page 277) (v)

Lunch: Italian Tuna Salad (page 279)
+ 1 portion of seasonal fruit

Supper: Cottage Pie (page 281)
+ 1 portion of seasonal fruit

Day 10

Breakfast: Egg Salad on Toast (page 291)
+ 1 portion of seasonal fruit

Lunch: Beet Hummus Salad (page 292) (v)
+ 1 portion of seasonal fruit

Supper: Leftover Cottage Pie (page 281) with
steamed greens + 1 portion of seasonal fruit

VEGAN MENU

Prep day recipes:

Beet Hummus (page 136)

Spiced Seed Sprinkle (page 140)

Nut Granola (page 141)

Day 1

Breakfast: Turmeric & Mango Spiced Chia Pot (page 148)

Lunch: Rainbow Abundance Bowl (page 151) + 1 portion of seasonal fruit

Supper: Puy Lentils with Roasted Vegetables (page 158), Cashew Nut Cream (page 159), and an arugula salad + 1 portion of seasonal fruit

Day 2:

Breakfast: Roasted Vegetables with Cashew Nut Cream on Toast (page 173) + 1 portion of seasonal fruit

Lunch: Walnut Lentil Pâté in lettuce cups (page 174) + 1 portion of seasonal fruit

Supper: Asian-style Salad with cashews (page 175) + 1 portion of seasonal fruit

Day 3

Breakfast: Banana, Mint & Lime Smoothie (page 182)

Lunch: Asian-style Salad with Mango (page 188)

Supper: Eggplant & Chickpea Curry (page 186) + 1 portion of seasonal fruit

Day 4

Breakfast: Overnight Oat Crumble with Apple (page 196)

Lunch: Leftover Eggplant & Chickpea Curry (page 186) + 1 portion of seasonal fruit

Supper: Smoked Tofu with Orange & Avocado Salsa (page 200)

Day 5

Breakfast: Overnight Oat Crumble with Berries (page 196)

Lunch: Roasted Vegetable Soup (page 210) +1 portion of seasonal fruit

Supper: Spicy Tomato & Lima Bean Zucchini Noodles (page 211) + 1 portion of seasonal fruit

The 10-Day Plan to Nourish & Glow

Day 6

Breakfast: Nut Granola with Berries (page 219)

Lunch: Kale Waldorf Salad (page 228)

Supper: Chopped Salad with Sweet Potato Fries (page 232) + Nutty Banana Nice Cream (page 227)

Day 7

Breakfast: Pea & Sweet Potato Fritter (page 246) + 1 portion of seasonal fruit

Lunch: Chopped Black Bean Salad (page 247)

Supper: Falafel Burgers with a portobello mushroom "bun" (page 248) + Nutty Chocolate Pot (page 245)

Day 8

Breakfast: Sweet Potato Toasts with Scrambled Tofu, roasted tomatoes, and kale (page 267) + 1 portion of seasonal fruit

Lunch: Falafel Salad (page 270) + 1 portion of seasonal fruit

Supper: Stuffed Peppers with Chili (page 262) + Baked Orange & Almond Pear (page 266)

Day 9

Breakfast: Baked Pear Breakfast Bowl (page 277)

Lunch: Green Bean, Pea & Pistachio Salad (page 282) + 1 portion of seasonal fruit

Supper: Lentil "Cottage" Pie (page 283) + 1 portion of seasonal fruit

Day 10

Breakfast: Coconut Quinoa Porridge (page 294)

Lunch: Beet Hummus & Avocado Toast (page 295) +1 portion of seasonal fruit

Supper: Leftover Lentil "Cottage" Pie with steamed greens (page 283) + 1 portion of seasonal fruit

PREPARATION DAY

This is the day to get your kitchen (and head!) cleared out and prepped for the next 10 days of healthy cooking and eating. I really encourage you to do this on a Saturday, if that is a less busy day of the week for you. Mondays are often the most challenging day to start something new, and so if Day 1 is a Sunday, you'll have had some time to prepare.

Set 3 or 4 hours aside to do your preparation for the week ahead. It might sound like a lot of time, but I promise it will in fact *save* you time throughout the week—and we are going to make those hours work hard. Have a good read through the instructions before you get going though, so you know where you are aiming. The idea is that you are preparing the next dish as the previous one cooks or cools.

Start with cleaning out and tidying your cupboards and fridge. If you share a home with others, then give them their own shelves and put any treats onto their shelves or cupboard. Create your own space for your food for the coming days. This is a great time to check what spices and seasonings you have and, if they are still fresh (they often aren't!), you can cross them off your shopping list for the 10-day plan. Make sure that it is an honest clearout—get rid of out-of-date foods, packages, and jars and all of the things that you know talk to you in weak moments.

Next, do a checklist of what you already have from the shopping list and cross it off. Then do your shopping—you can either do it every few days, or order everything for the first week of the plan.

I really encourage a good clearout of the kitchen. Get your surfaces clean and clear and ready for some quality time in there! And maybe even clear out your drawers, donate pans that you never use (I did this recently; it is so weird how much stuff we hang on to), and check that you have garbage bags and storage containers. Clear out your fridge and make space in the freezer.

My best tip is to start with a clean kitchen and an empty dishwasher. Throw dirty bowls and utensils straight into the dishwasher as you go along to help keep your kitchen clean and tidy.

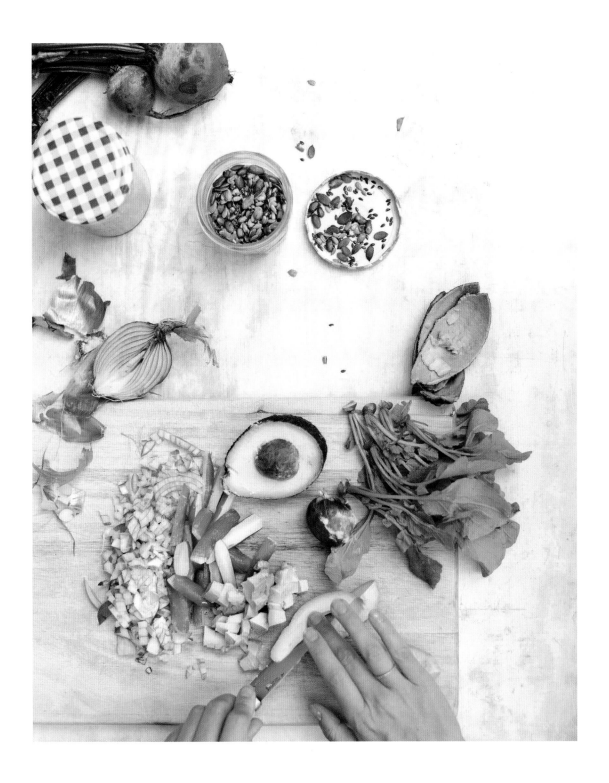

Preparation day cooking

- Beet Hummus
- Nut Granola
- Spiced Seed Sprinkle
- Turmeric & Mango Spiced Chia Pot
- Vegetable preparation for the next couple of days

If you are slightly less confident in the kitchen, here is a suggested breakdown of your prep day cooking. However, if you are a keen cook, you may not need this! All recipes are written in full in the following pages.

PREP DAY STEP-BY-STEP INSTRUCTIONS

1. Preheat the oven to 350°F.

2. Make sure you have all your ingredients and equipment on hand.

3. Wash the beets and wrap them in aluminum foil, then roast them in the oven following the recipe on page 136. I set a timer for 60 minutes to remind me to check them.

4. While the beets are cooking, you can start to make the Nut Granola following the recipe on page 141. Once the granola is spread out onto a parchment paper-lined baking tray, place to one side.

5. Next, prepare the Spiced Seed Sprinkle according to the recipe on page 140. Spread out onto another parchment paper-lined baking tray.

6. Place both the granola and spiced seeds into the oven (they cook at the same temperature).

7. Set another timer for 10 minutes. When it goes off, stir both mixtures around, and then put them both back into the oven for a further 10 minutes. Keep a watchful eye throughout this second half of cooking—they can burn easily in powerful ovens, so you may find they only need another 7–8 minutes. Once done, take them out and leave to cool completely.

8. While the granola and spiced seeds are baking, you can get on with making the Turmeric & Mango Spiced Chia Pot for breakfast tomorrow. Follow the recipe on page 148. I find making it in a jam jar with a secure lid is easiest. Once they are made, you can just put them straight into the fridge.

9. When the 60-minute timer goes off, check on your beets. If they are cooked then they will be tender to the point of a knife. If they are still a bit hard, then put them back into the oven, set your timer for another 10 minutes, and then re-check. Once done, leave them to cool.

10. By now you should have everything out of the oven, and a kitchen full of delicious smells! The oven can therefore be turned off.

11. When the beets are cool enough to handle, unwrap the foil and peel. Use some to complete the recipe for Beet Hummus (see page 136). Once made, divide the mixture into 3. Save one portion of this for your lunch tomorrow, and put the remaining 2 portions into the freezer for another day. I tend to use old yogurt containers or similar for this, wrapping the tops well before freezing them.

12. The leftover beets can be placed, covered, into the fridge for later in the week.

13. Once the spiced seeds and granola are completely cool, put them into separate airtight jars and store somewhere cool (although they don't need to go into the fridge).

14. If you can face it after all this preparation, the icing on the cake would be to get ahead and prepare your lunch for tomorrow—a wonderfully colorful Rainbow Abundance Bowl (see page 151).

15. If you're following the vegan plan, soak the cashews to make your Cashew Nut Cream for supper tomorrow (see page 159).

BEET HUMMUS (V)

MAKES: 3 portions

PYRAMID: **1**

I absolutely love hummus! It's a delicious way to get extra fiber, plant protein, healthy fats, and calcium (especially from the tahini) into my diet, plus I never get bored with it as there are so many different flavor possibilities.

This recipe makes a very generous amount, but it freezes well and works out much more economical than buying it at the supermarket.

If you are following the meal plan, it's a good idea to roast all the beets you'll need for the next few days at the same time, in which case, you will need 2–3 medium raw beets—then just follow the recipe as below to roast them together. You will use these extra beets to make a delicious soup later in the week. If you are strapped for time, however, you can use pre-cooked ones from the supermarket instead.

1 medium raw beet (about 7 oz) (2–3 medium beets if you are following the meal plan)

¼ cup chopped fresh or 2 teaspoons dried dill

1 clove of garlic, peeled

1 x 14 oz can of chickpeas, drained and rinsed

3 tablespoons tahini

½ teaspoon salt

juice and zest of 1 lemon

Preheat the oven to 350°F.

Wrap the whole beets individually in small squares of foil lined with parchment paper and place on a tray in the oven for 60–90 minutes (the baking time will vary depending on the size of the beet), or until a sharp knife slips easily into the center. I usually do this when I have something else in the oven.

When cool enough to handle, use paper towel to slip the skin off the beets (see tip opposite).

Place one peeled beet in the food processor along with any juices in the foil and the dill. Add all the other hummus ingredients. Blend for 3–4 minutes, until really smooth. You may need to add a tiny splash of cold water if your mixture is looking very thick. Taste and adjust the seasoning as necessary.

Keep about a third of the mixture in a small container in the fridge (to make your vibrant Rainbow Abundance Bowl for lunch tomorrow, see page 151). Freeze the remaining portions individually.

TIP: When handling beets, use a little olive oil as you would use hand cream to form a skin barrier, then hold the beets with paper towel and the skins should slip off easily, without staining your hands.

VARIATIONS

Using the hummus base ingredients (garlic, chickpeas, tahini, salt, and lemon), add your choice of the following flavor combinations before blitzing in your food processor.

- Paprika: 1 teaspoon paprika/smoked paprika

- Traditional: 1 teaspoon ground cumin and ½ teaspoon ground coriander

- Green: a handful of arugula

- Pesto: ½ a bunch of fresh basil (stems removed), 2 tablespoons olive oil, 2 tablespoons pine nuts

- Parsley: ½ a bunch of fresh parsley (stems removed) and 1 teaspoon lemon zest

- Guacamole: ½ a ripe avocado, extra zest and juice of ½ a lemon, ¼ of a bunch of fresh cilantro leaves, ½ teaspoon chili powder (optional)

- Tomato: 3–4 sun-dried tomatoes (drained of their oil)

- Olive: 3 tablespoons pitted black or green olives and 1 tablespoon olive oil

- Carrot and cilantro: 2 roasted carrots (great if you have them as leftovers after Sunday lunch), with 1 teaspoon ground coriander and ¼ of a bunch of cilantro

- Curried: 1 teaspoon garam masala, ½ teaspoon turmeric, ½ teaspoon ground cumin, 1 teaspoon tomato puree, 1 teaspoon fresh ginger (peeled and grated)

- Red pepper and walnut: 1 roasted red pepper (seeds and stems removed) and 2 tablespoons of chopped walnuts

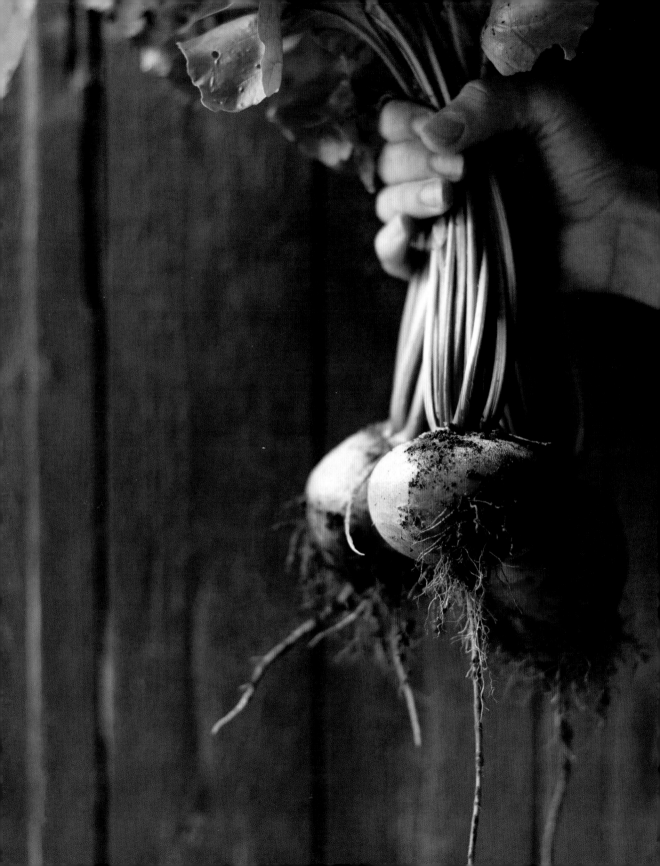

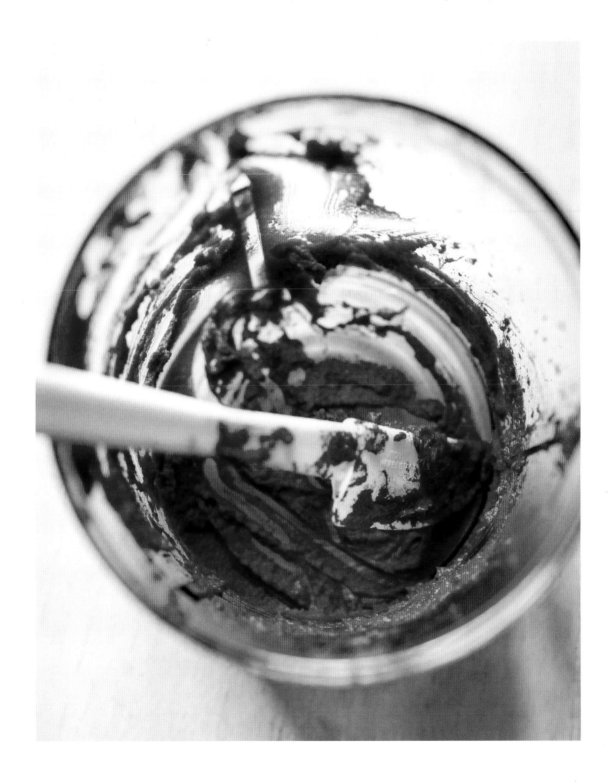

SPICED SEED SPRINKLE (V)

MAKES: 6 portions • 1 portion = 1 oz / about 2–3 tablespoons

PYRAMID: / / 1

You can buy packages of flavored toasted seeds in supermarkets and health-food shops, but at great expense, and I always think a homemade version tastes better. It's great to have a jar of them in the cupboard, to throw on top of soups or salads. I like a mix of pumpkin, flaxseed, and sunflower seeds, but feel free to use whatever you like—or indeed, have in your cupboard! You can always play around with the flavors too—I sometimes make them using a harissa spice mix, or paprika, which is equally delicious, so feel free to use whatever herbs and spices you have lying around.

6 oz mixed seeds

1 teaspoon light olive oil

¼ teaspoon chili powder, or 1 teaspoon curry powder

a generous pinch of sea salt and a few grinds of black pepper

Preheat the oven to 350°F.

Combine all the ingredients in a bowl and mix well together. Spread out thinly on a parchment paper-lined baking sheet and bake for 10 minutes. Stir, then bake for a further 7–10 minutes. Watch them carefully though, during the second half of the cooking—they can burn quickly, depending on the strength of your oven. Remove once they are golden brown.

Allow to cool completely and store in an airtight container for up to 10 days.

NOTE: One portion could be counted as any one of the Positive Nutrition Pyramid food groups above.

NUT GRANOLA (V)

MAKES: 4–6 portions

PYRAMID: / / 1

Nuts are nature's powerhouses. This grain-free granola recipe is a perfect way to enjoy them.

It's great to have in your cupboard for adding to fruit or yogurt for a quick breakfast, and keeps well in an airtight container for 10 days or so. Just try to avoid getting into the habit of eating it directly from the jar like one member of my team does . . . !

6 oz roughly chopped mixed nuts (unsalted)

1 tablespoon coconut oil or light olive oil

1 tablespoon sweetener of choice (such as honey/maple syrup/coconut sugar)

½ teaspoon organic vanilla extract

a pinch of sea salt flakes

1 teaspoon cinnamon

zest of 1 orange (optional)

Preheat the oven to 350°F.

Roughly chop the nuts (or pulse a few times in a blender).

Combine all the ingredients in a bowl and tip onto a large baking tray lined with parchment paper. Bake for 20 minutes, stirring halfway through.

Allow to cool completely, then store in an airtight container.

NOTE: One portion could be counted as any one of the Positive Nutrition Pyramid food groups above.

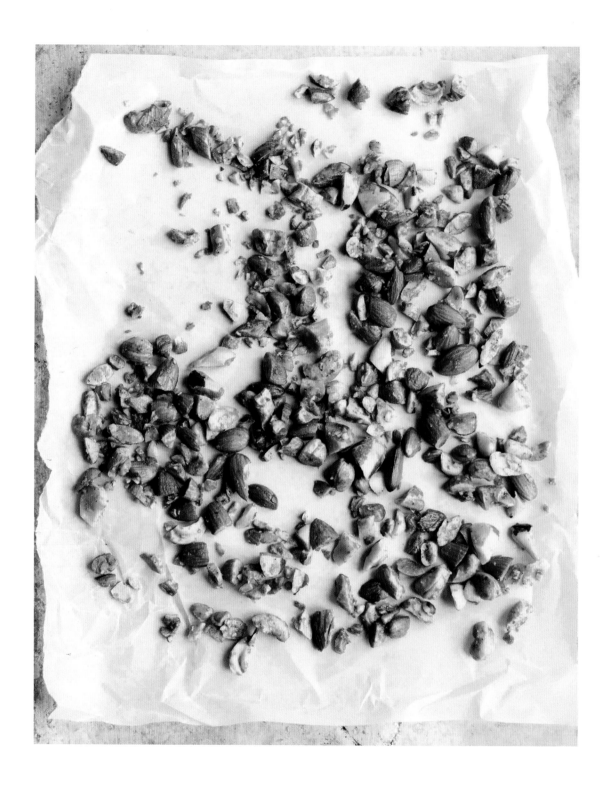

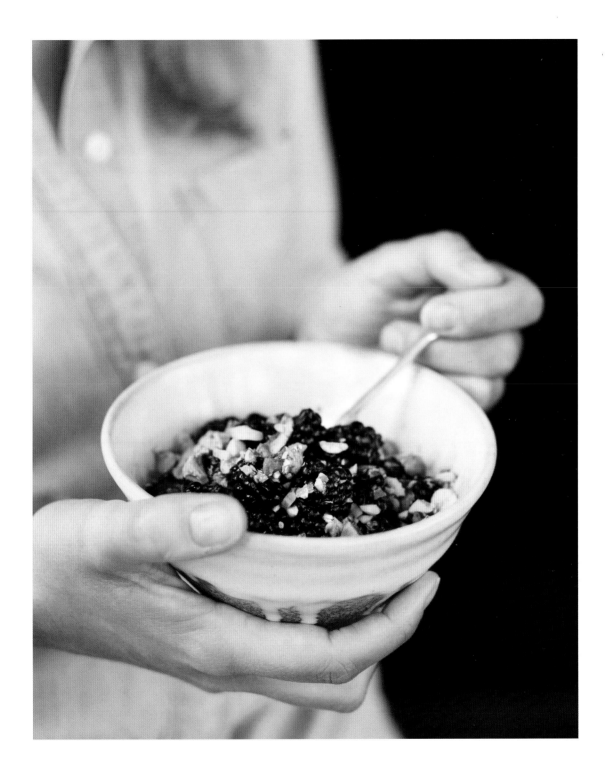

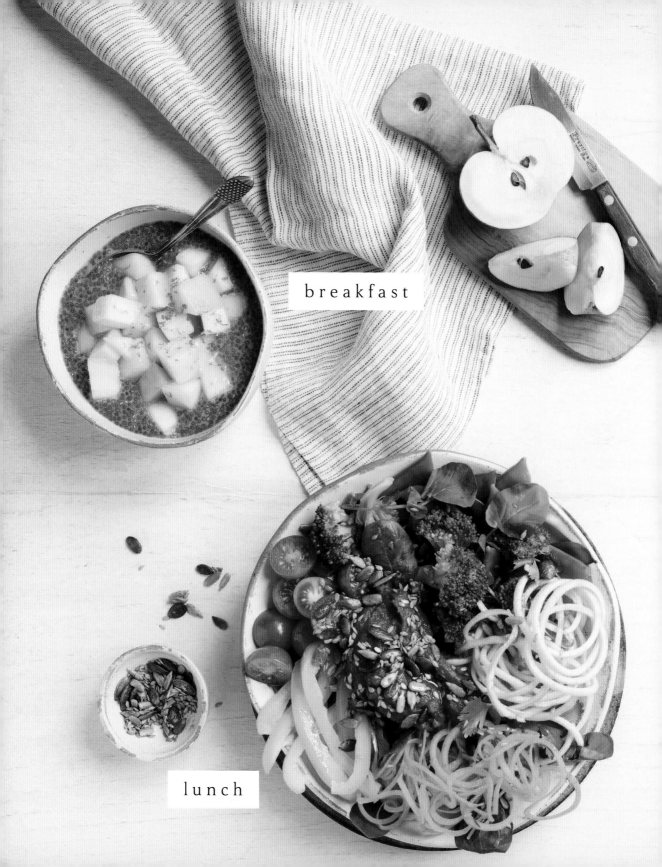

breakfast

lunch

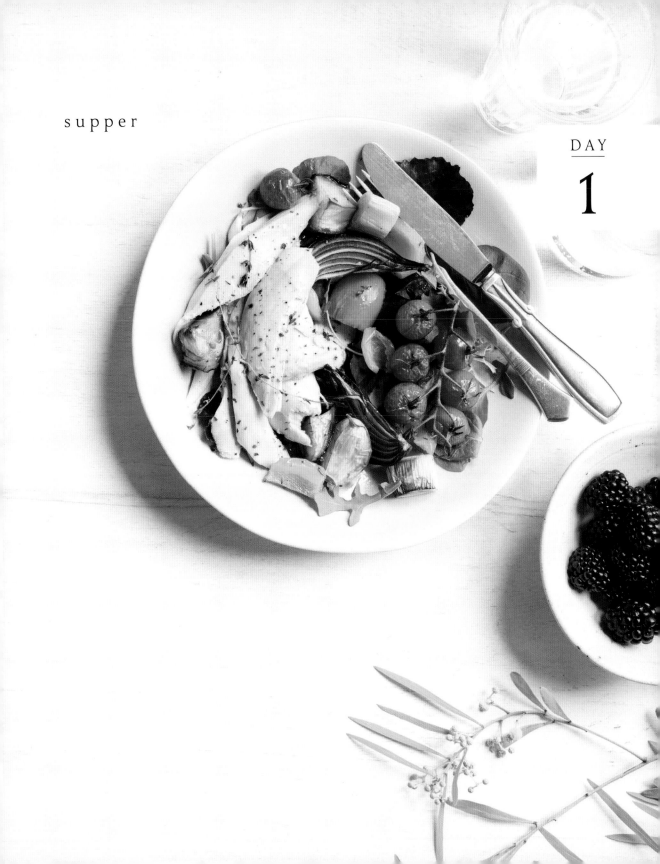

supper

DAY 1

BREAKFAST: TURMERIC & MANGO SPICED CHIA POT (v)

LUNCH: RAINBOW ABUNDANCE BOWL (v)
+ 1 PORTION OF SEASONAL FRUIT

SUPPER: ROAST CHICKEN with ROASTED VEGETABLES
+ 1 PORTION OF SEASONAL FRUIT

vegan alternatives:

SUPPER: PUY LENTILS with ROASTED VEGETABLES,
CASHEW NUT CREAM, and an ARUGULA SALAD
+ 1 PORTION OF SEASONAL FRUIT

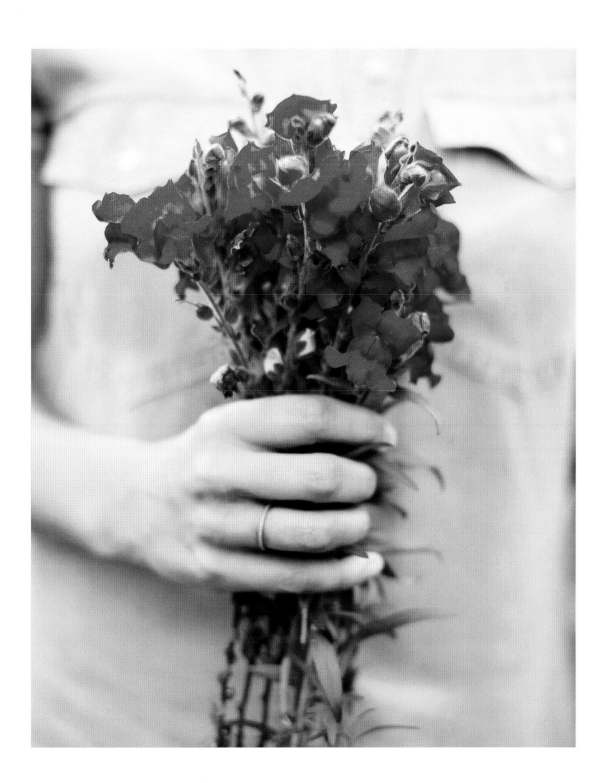

TURMERIC & MANGO
SPICED CHIA POT (V)

PYRAMID:

This is such an easy breakfast or dessert. Chia seeds provide some healthy omega-3 fats, fiber, protein, and multiple other nutrients. And they don't require any cooking—just soak them in any type of liquid, add some fruit or flavor, and enjoy. I do find that mixing them with a creamy milk like coconut is best (from a carton, not a can) and helps to take away the slightly slimy texture that freaks some people out! This breakfast is suitable for vegans too.

¾ cup unsweetened coconut milk (from a carton)

¼ level teaspoon ground turmeric

½ teaspoon ground cinnamon

¼ teaspoon ground cardamom

¼ teaspoon ground cloves

1 Medjool date, chopped, or 1 teaspoon sweetener of your choice

3 tablespoons chia seeds

½ to ¾ cup mango, diced

zest of ½ a lime

Whizz everything except the chia seeds, mango, and lime zest in a blender. If you don't have a blender, you can just whisk the coconut milk and spices together, then stir in the chopped dates or sweetener.

Add the chia seeds, mix thoroughly, then pour the mixture into a small glass or jam jar, and top with the fruit and lime zest

Leave in the fridge to set overnight. I like to add a little squeeze of the lime before serving for a zingy hit.

You are likely to have some mango left over from making this recipe. If you are following the main plan, then this would be a tasty portion of fruit for one of your meals. If you are following the vegan plan, however, you will use the leftover mango to create a delicious Asian-inspired salad a little later in the week—so wrap it well and keep it in the fridge for then.

NOTE: If you don't have all these spices already, you can substitute 1 level teaspoon of pumpkin pie spice for the ground cinnamon, cardamom, and cloves.

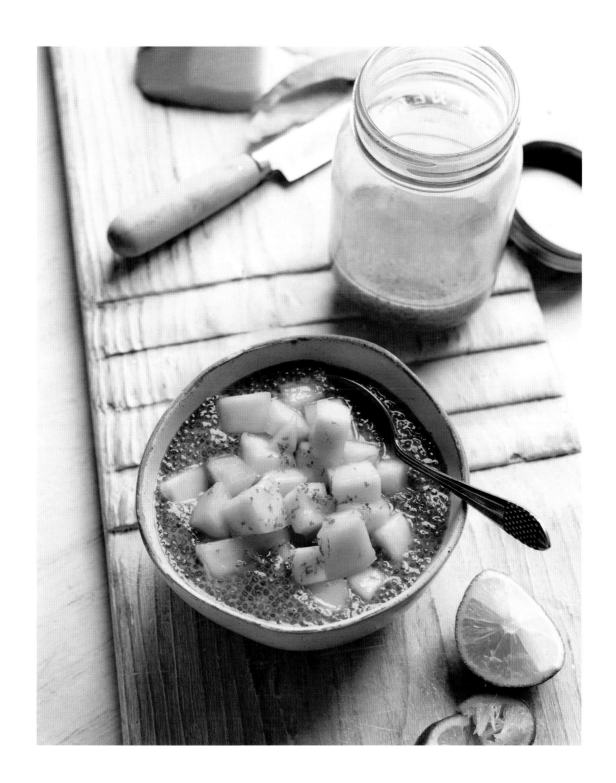

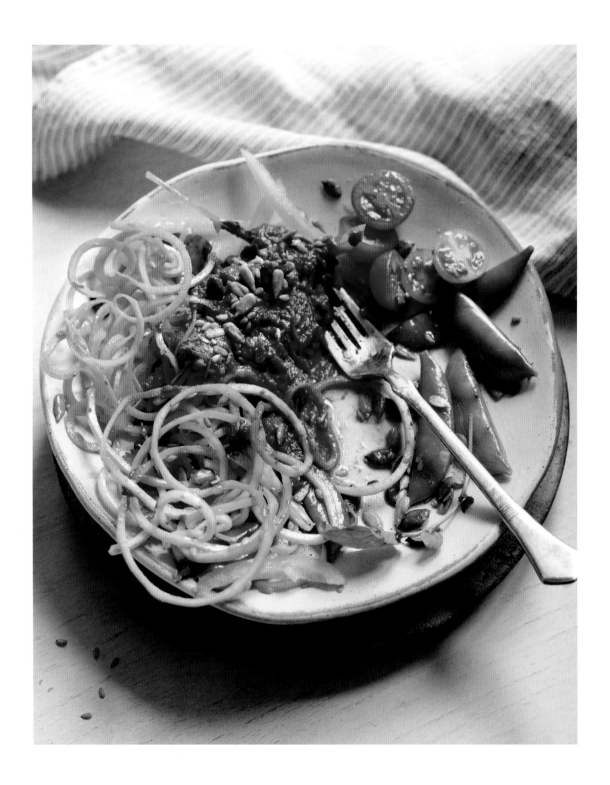

RAINBOW ABUNDANCE BOWL (V)

7 oz sugar snap peas, blanched or steamed and refreshed

7 oz broccoli (about 1 small head), blanched or steamed and refreshed

1 small carrot, peeled and spiralized (or grated)

1 very small green or yellow zucchini, washed and spiralized (or grated)

6–8 cherry tomatoes, washed and halved

½ a yellow or orange pepper, seeded and cut into thin strips

1 handful of salad leaves of your choice, washed if necessary

1 portion of Beet Hummus (see page 136)

2–3 tablespoons Spiced Seed Sprinkle (see page 140)

a drizzle of extra-virgin olive oil

PYRAMID: 6

This is a big bowl of happiness to me! It's very filling and each mouthful is different. I love hummus with bowls of veggies and salad, and the garishly pink color of this beet version is unashamedly joyful.

I've doubled up the portions of steamed broccoli and sugar snap peas here—this means that you've got some ready to go for another meal later in the week. This recipe is suitable for vegans too.

———————————

Steam or blanch your sugar snap peas and broccoli for a few minutes, then refresh them in cold water. Once cooled, put half of these, covered, into the fridge—you will use them again for supper on Day 3.

Pat the remaining sugar snap peas and broccoli dry, and arrange with the rest of the vegetables in a bowl or lunch container. All of this can be prepared ahead of time and left in the fridge overnight.

Before serving, top your salad with a generous dollop of hummus, add a sprinkle of seed mix and a drizzle of extra-virgin olive oil, and enjoy!

ROAST CHICKEN with ROASTED VEGETABLES

FOR THE CHICKEN
(makes 4 generous portions, plus Chicken Stock, see page 156)

2 onions, peeled and halved

2 carrots, peeled and halved lengthwise

1 head of garlic, cut in half around the circumference

1 x 3 lb high-quality chicken

1 lemon, halved

½ a bunch of fresh thyme or a sprig of rosemary (optional)

sea salt and freshly ground black pepper

FOR THE ROASTED VEGETABLES
(makes 3 portions)

½ an eggplant, cut into 1-inch chunks (you'll use the other half later in the week)

1 red pepper, cut into chunks

½ a yellow or orange pepper, cut into chunks (use the other half from your Rainbow Abundance Bowl)

PYRAMID:

Roast chicken is one of my all-time favorite meals. I know it is hardly an original recipe, but sometimes having a simple, comforting dish up your sleeve is exactly what is needed. And this method allows you to really eke every last morsel of goodness out of a whole chicken, which helps justify the cost of going for the best bird you can find. I try to buy only organic chickens (both for health and animal welfare reasons), but if this is not possible, look for the highest-quality free-range option you can find instead.

———————————————

Preheat the oven to 400°F.

Place 3 onion halves, the carrots, and half the garlic bulb in the bottom of a roasting dish. Stuff the cavity of the chicken with the other half of the garlic bulb, the last onion half, and half the lemon, plus the thyme or sprig of rosemary if you are using them.

Place the chicken upside down on the vegetables (this will help to keep it super-moist during cooking) and season with salt and pepper. Pour water into the bottom of the tray to a depth of ½ an inch or so, then place in the oven and cook for 45 minutes.

1 red onion, peeled
and cut into 8 wedges

a large handful of cherry
tomatoes

1 small leek,
cut into 1-inch lengths

2 cloves of garlic,
peeled and sliced

light olive oil

sea salt and freshly ground
black pepper

1 teaspoon dried mixed herbs
(or if you have them, a few
extra sprigs of fresh thyme)

TO SERVE
(for supper tonight)

1 handful of mixed salad
leaves of your choice
(or steamed greens
if you'd prefer)

a little extra-virgin olive oil
and balsamic vinegar
if you like it

While the chicken is in the oven, chop your vegetables and garlic and place them on the widest baking tray you have so that they overlap as little as possible. Drizzle generously with olive oil, and sprinkle with salt, pepper, and the dried mixed herbs or thyme.

Put the vegetables into the oven when the chicken has been cooking for 45 minutes, and lower the heat to 325°F. Cook the chicken and vegetables together for a further 30 minutes. Take the chicken out when the juices run clear when the thigh is pierced and there is no hint of pink. Leave it to rest uncovered.

When the chicken has rested for 10–20 minutes, remove the roast vegetables from the oven. Keep an eye on the vegetables near the end of the cooking time, as depending on how you've chopped them, they may be done sooner. They should be tender and slightly brown at the edges.

Carve the chicken, and serve yourself about a quarter of its meat (around 5 oz), about a third of the roasted vegetables and a big handful of salad leaves of your choice (or steamed greens in winter if you prefer). You might like to add a drizzle of olive oil and balsamic vinegar over your salad for extra flavor.

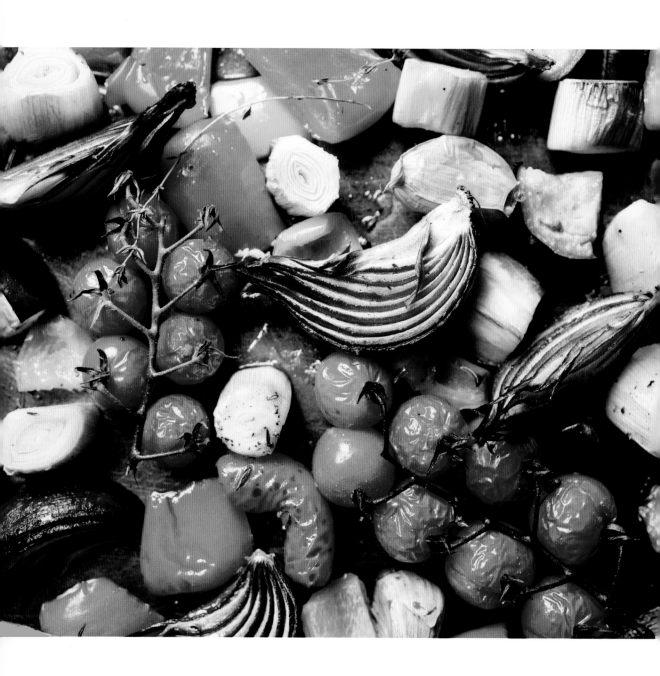

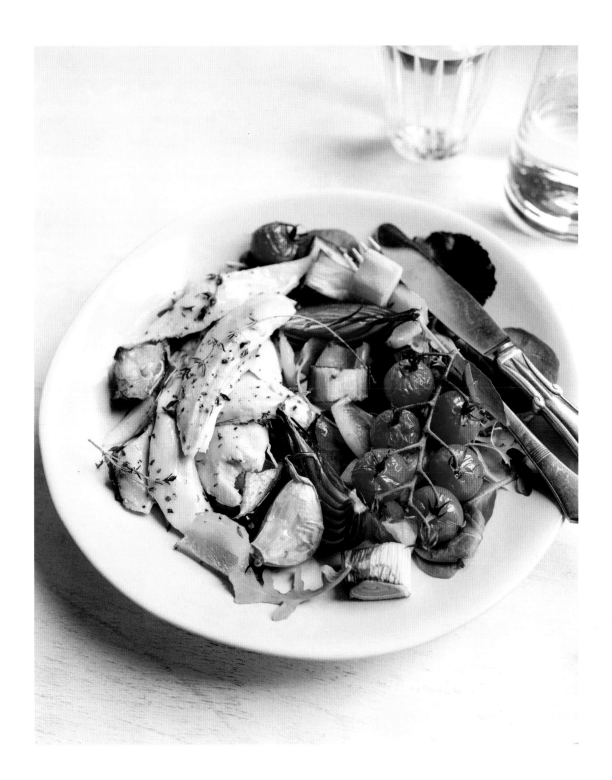

CHICKEN STOCK

Making stock from leftover chicken bones and veggies isn't as hard as you might imagine—just boil it all slowly to extract every last ounce of goodness. It becomes a beautiful golden liquid, which can either be enjoyed on its own, or added as a base to soups, stews, and casseroles. There are two methods explained here, depending on whether or not you have a slow cooker. I highly recommend investing in one if you can.

FROM THE ROAST CHICKEN
RECIPE *(see page 152)*

the chicken bones

the trivet vegetables
(carrots, onions, garlic)

the pan liquid

1 leek, roughly chopped

2 carrots, peeled

1 stick of celery

6 black peppercorns

a few sprigs of thyme

STOVETOP METHOD

Break up the chicken carcass and place it in your deepest, biggest pot. Add any of the smaller bones, skin, trivet vegetables, and juices from the pan. Throw in the leek, carrots, celery, peppercorns, and thyme. Pour in enough cold water to cover, plus an extra inch.

Bring the pot to a boil then turn down to the lowest possible heat (you might need to move the pot to your smallest element to reduce the heat even more), cover with a tight-fitting lid, and leave to simmer for as long as you can—ideally 4–5 hours (although you can get away with 2–3 hours if you're pressed for time).

SLOW COOKER METHOD

Put all the ingredients into your slow cooker, cover completely with water, and turn on to low.

Leave to cook overnight.

ONCE COOKED

Strain through a sieve into a heatproof bowl, and leave to cool completely in the fridge. This allows the fat to separate and rise to the top, so that you can then remove it with a spoon.

It will be used to make a curry (see page 186) and a soup (see page 206) later in the plan.

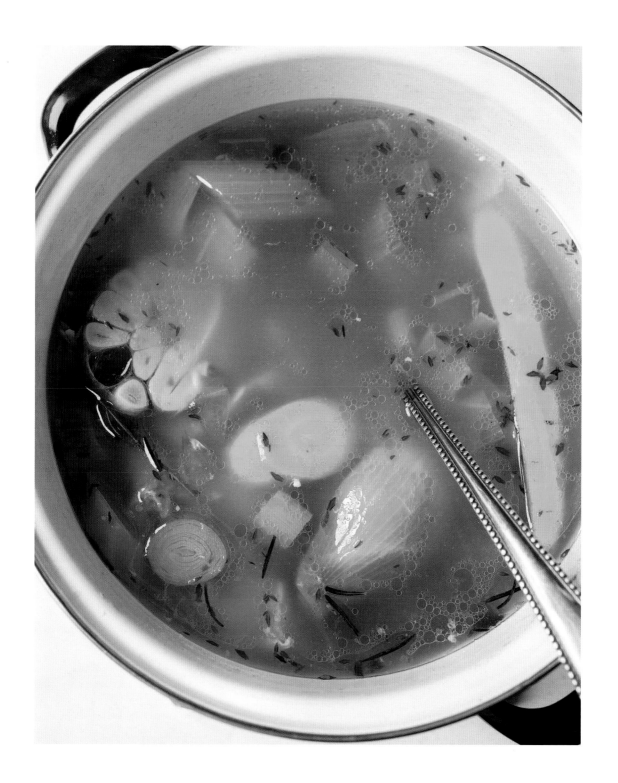

VEGAN ALTERNATIVES

PUY LENTILS with ROASTED VEGETABLES (V)

MAKES: 3 portions

½ a large eggplant, cut into 1-inch chunks (you'll use the other half later in the week)

1 red pepper, cut into chunks

1 yellow pepper, cut into chunks

1 red onion, peeled and cut into 8 wedges

a large handful of cherry tomatoes

1 small leek, cut into 1-inch lengths

2 cloves of garlic, peeled and sliced

light olive oil

1 teaspoon dried mixed herbs

½ a bunch of fresh thyme, leaves removed and chopped

sea salt and freshly ground black pepper, to taste

TO SERVE

generous ¾ cup ready-cooked Puy lentils

4 sun-dried tomatoes, drained and chopped

PYRAMID:

This classic combination of roasted Mediterranean vegetables, dark speckles of protein-packed Puy lentils, and some tangy sun-dried tomatoes definitely has an air of Italy about it! I tend to cheat a bit when it comes to cooking lentils, and often buy the ready-cooked pouches (available at most big supermarkets).

Preheat the oven to 350°F.

Chop your vegetables and garlic and place them on the widest baking tray you have so that they overlap as little as possible. Drizzle generously with olive oil, then sprinkle with the dried herbs and fresh thyme. Season with salt and pepper.

Roast for 45–55 minutes (depending on the strength of your oven and the size of the vegetable pieces). They should be tender and slightly brown at the edges.

DAY 1 • Vegan Supper

1 tablespoon tomato puree

1 tablespoon chopped fresh parsley

1 tablespoon chopped fresh basil

1 portion of Cashew Nut Cream (see below)

a big handful of arugula leaves

While the vegetables are cooking, you may wish to prepare the Cashew Nut Cream.

Once the vegetables are done, place a third in a saucepan.

Add the lentils, sun-dried tomatoes and tomato puree, and a splash of water and place over low–medium heat.

Gently warm through for a few minutes, stirring regularly, then mix through the parsley and basil. Season to taste. Serve with Cashew Nut Cream and a handful of arugula.

CASHEW NUT CREAM (V)

MAKES: 2 portions

PYRAMID: 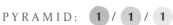 1 / 1 / 1

This wonderful sauce is dairy-free heaven and goes beautifully with dishes that might traditionally have benefited from something a little creamy!

½ cup cashews, soaked in ½ cup water (ideally overnight or for at least 3 hours)

juice of ½ a lemon

1 tablespoon extra-virgin olive oil

1 tablespoon nutritional yeast flakes

a pinch of salt

3–4 tablespoons cold water

Drain the cashews from their soaking water, then whizz in a high-speed blender (a NutriBullet works well) with the rest of the ingredients. Scrape down the edges of the blender a couple of times, to make sure everything is well incorporated.

Depending on the nuts and your blender, you may need to adjust the water, adding a little extra bit by bit until you have your desired consistency. It should be like thick yogurt.

NOTE: One portion could be counted as any one of the Positive Nutrition Pyramid food groups above.

COMPLETE TODAY'S PREPARATION

after supper

1. Strip the remaining chicken meat from the bones. Add the bones to a pot and cover with water, to make your Chicken Stock (see page 156).

2. Separate the leftover roast chicken into 3 portions. Use one portion to make the Chicken Pâté (see page 168) for lunch tomorrow, and refrigerate the rest.

3. You could also make the Breakfast Frittata for tomorrow morning now (see page 167), leaving it in the fridge overnight.

4. Leave the rest of the roasted vegetables in the fridge for now, ready to make a soup later on in the plan.

for the vegan plan

1. *Make the Walnut Lentil Pâté for lunch for tomorrow (see page 174).*

2. *Leave one portion of roasted vegetables, covered, in the fridge with half the Cashew Nut Cream for breakfast tomorrow.*

3. *Leave the remaining portion of roasted vegetables in the fridge for now, ready to make a soup later on in the plan.*

Mindful Moment

You may find that steering clear of snacking and perhaps eating different food than normal has led to some strong cravings. So tomorrow's mindful moment is to pay attention to these— instead of just trying to ignore them.

So if you get any cravings during the course of the day, or indeed throughout the rest of the meal plan, try to take a moment to pay full and complete attention to them. What *specifically* is it that you are craving? How are you feeling right now? Is this a new or a normal craving for you?

Take a moment to reassure yourself that cravings are completely normal, and that hunger is really not something to be scared of. It is helpful to feel moderately hungry in the lead-up to a meal, especially if you are not used to eating this sort of food.

If you find the cravings persist, try to find a distracting activity and drink a large glass of water. And don't forget . . .

"Nobody has ever died from starvation between nourishing meals!"

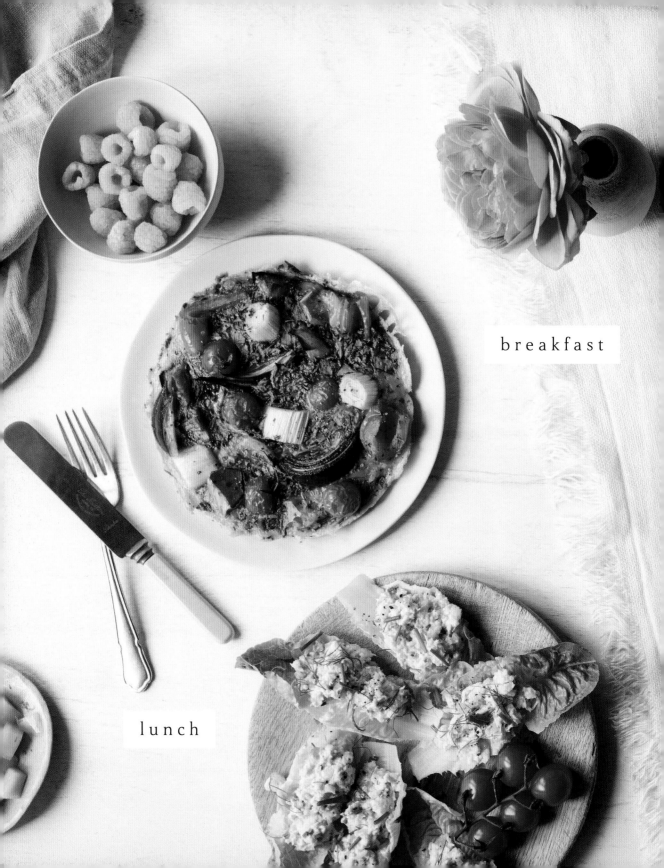

breakfast

lunch

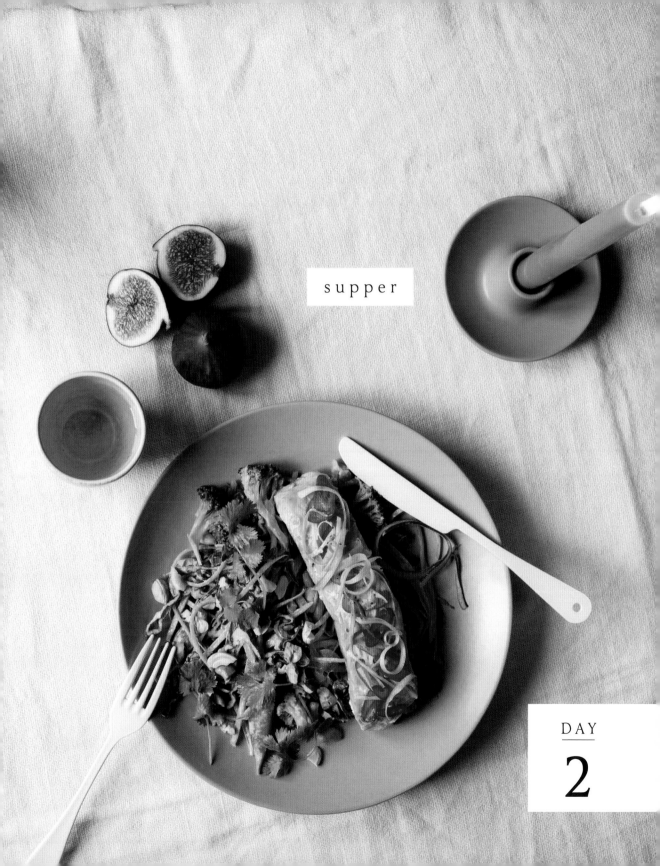

supper

DAY 2

BREAKFAST: BREAKFAST FRITTATA
+ 1 PORTION of SEASONAL FRUIT

LUNCH: CHICKEN PÂTÉ in LETTUCE CUPS
+ 1 PORTION of SEASONAL FRUIT

SUPPER: WILD SALMON PARCELS
with ASIAN-STYLE SALAD
+ 1 PORTION of SEASONAL FRUIT

---

vegan alternatives:

BREAKFAST: ROASTED VEGETABLES with
CASHEW NUT CREAM on TOAST
+ 1 PORTION of SEASONAL FRUIT

LUNCH: WALNUT LENTIL PÂTÉ in LETTUCE CUPS
+ 1 PORTION of SEASONAL FRUIT

SUPPER: ASIAN-STYLE SALAD with CASHEWS
+ 1 PORTION of SEASONAL FRUIT

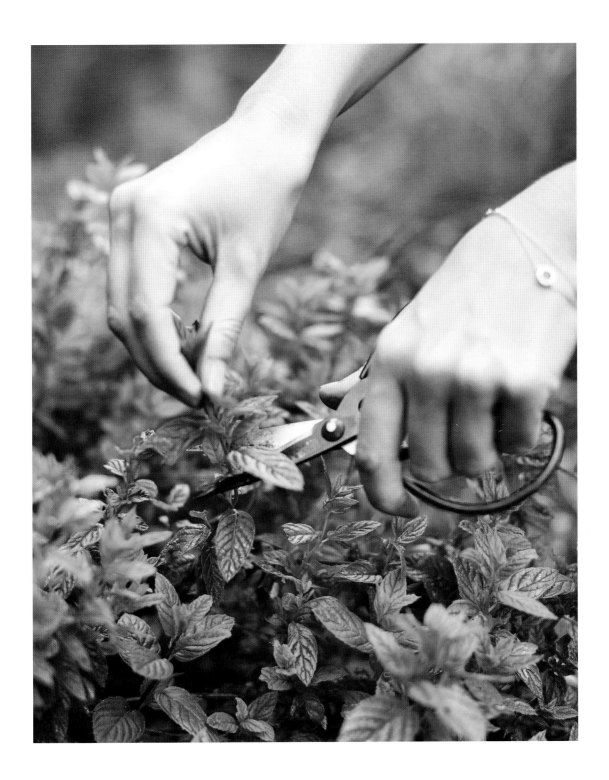

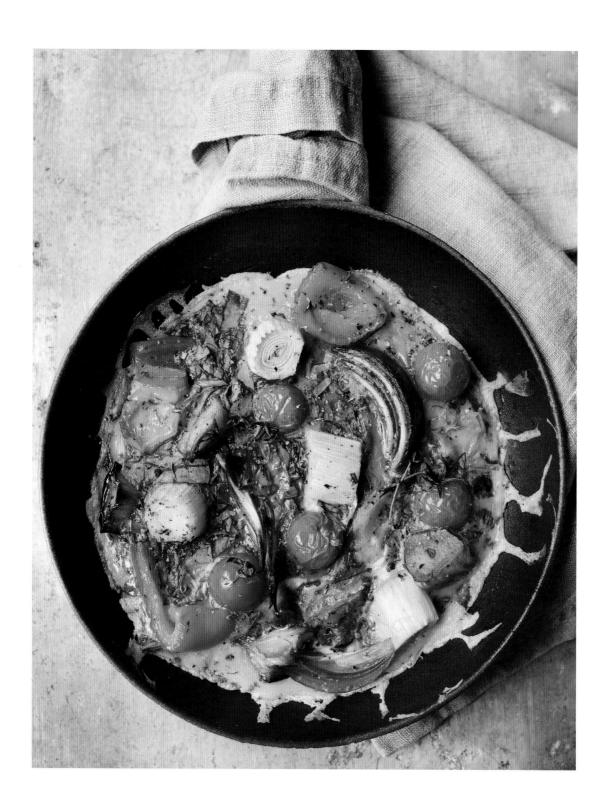

BREAKFAST FRITTATA

PYRAMID:

Eggs are my go-to for a quick, filling meal, and whipping them up into a frittata is a great way to use up any leftover vegetables. Eggs are an excellent source of protein and healthy fats, as well as 18 other essential nutrients (such as magnesium, zinc, iodine, vitamin A, and vitamin E). It has become common to worry about eating too many eggs because of their fat and cholesterol content; however, the cholesterol in eggs actually has a very limited effect on blood cholesterol levels, so enjoying up to around 6 per week is generally considered absolutely fine.

If you find the frittata gets a little dry after being in the fridge, try adding a dollop of pesto or a dash of Tabasco to liven it up. You can warm it up before eating if you wish, but I enjoy it just as much cold. It's also an excellent meal to take when traveling as it doesn't drip or spill.

1 teaspoon light olive oil or coconut oil

1 portion of leftover roasted vegetables

1 handful of spinach, washed and finely chopped

2 large eggs, preferably free-range or organic, whisked

sea salt and freshly ground black pepper, to taste

1 teaspoon dried oregano or mixed herbs, to taste

Preheat the broiler to hot (425°F), and place a rack near the very top of your oven.

In a small frying pan, heat 1 teaspoon of oil over low heat (you might not need much oil, as the roasted vegetables should already be well coated) and add all the vegetables and the spinach. Mix well to prevent any bits sticking and burning.

Whisk the eggs with some salt, pepper, and oregano or mixed herbs and evenly pour the mixture over the vegetables. Shake the pan back and forth to even the egg mixture out.

After 2–3 minutes on the burner over the lowest heat, put your frittata under the broiler to finish for another 3–4 minutes, or until cooked all the way through. Make sure it doesn't burn!

Allow to cool completely in the pan (this will help stop it falling apart as you remove it). Slide a rubber spatula around the pan to help ease it away from the edges before flipping it out onto a plate. If making ahead, store in the fridge overnight.

CHICKEN PÂTÉ

5 oz leftover roast chicken

1 stick of celery, diced

1 scallion, finely sliced

zest and juice of ½ a lemon

½ teaspoon chopped
fresh dill

½ teaspoon chopped
fresh chives

sea salt and freshly ground
black pepper, to taste

2 tablespoons dairy-free
coconut yogurt (or full-fat
organic mayonnaise)

TO SERVE

1 Bibb lettuce

a handful of cherry tomatoes

PYRAMID:

I read a recipe for Gwyneth Paltrow's favorite chicken salad on goop.com a few months ago and it swiftly became mine too. I've played around with the flavors and this is now my favorite version—such a good way to use up leftover chicken, which can go a bit dry. I love to make a sort of sandwich with lettuce cups.

Put the chicken into a blender and pulse four or five times. Add the celery and pulse twice more. Pour into a bowl and stir in the other ingredients, mixing well. If making ahead, pack into an airtight container and refrigerate for lunch tomorrow.

To serve, scoop the chicken pâté into the lettuce cups and enjoy alongside a handful of cherry tomatoes.

TIPS: If you can't get hold of fresh herbs, you can replace them with 1 teaspoon of dried mixed herbs.

If stringy celery bothers you, peel the outside.

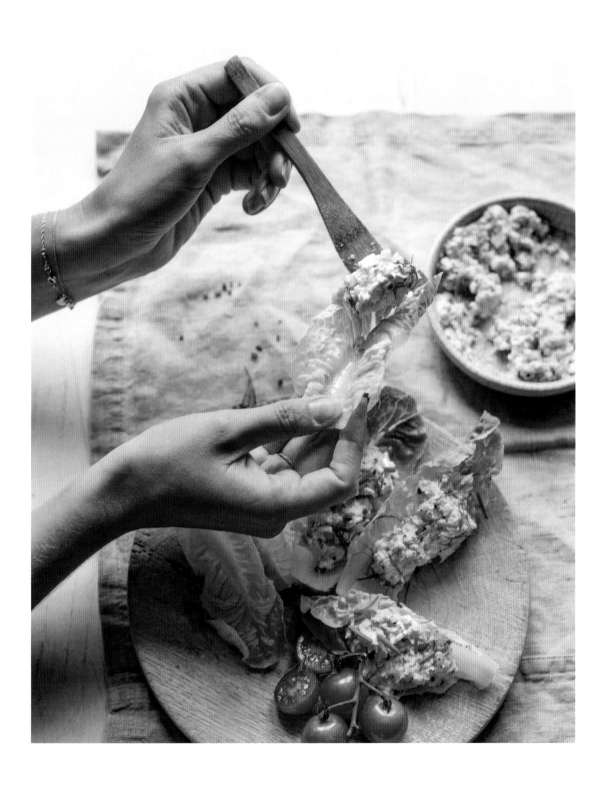

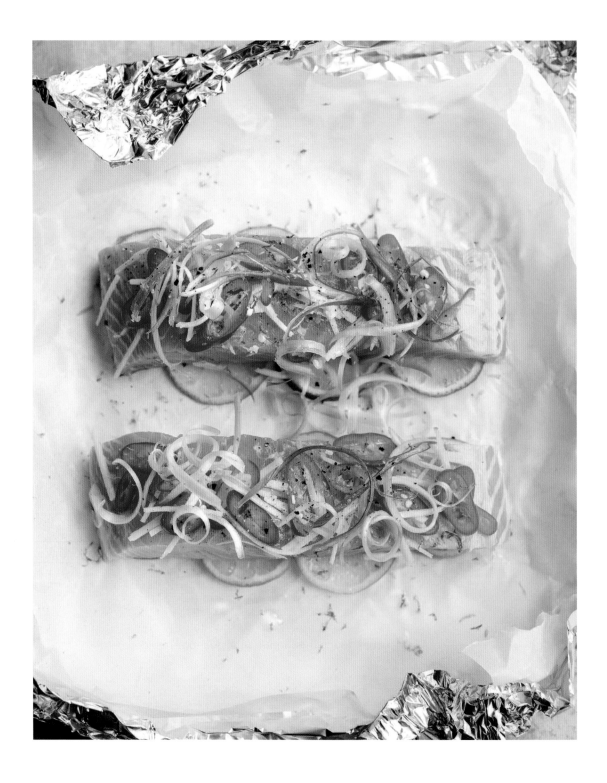

WILD SALMON PARCELS with ASIAN-STYLE SALAD

FOR THE ASIAN-STYLE SALAD
(makes 2 portions)

½ a small head of red cabbage, finely sliced

2 medium carrots, peeled and julienned or grated

½ a bunch of cilantro, stalks removed, leaves chopped

zest of 1 lime

3 cups leftover steamed broccoli, sliced

1 cup leftover sugar snap peas

scant ¼ cup cashews

FOR THE SALMON PARCELS
(makes 2 portions)

1 lime, zested and then sliced

2 wild salmon fillets (one for next day)

about ½-inch piece of ginger peeled and grated

2 scallions, chopped

1 mild chili pepper, sliced (optional)

2 teaspoons olive oil

freshly ground black pepper

PYRAMID:

Making fish parcels is such a lovely, easy way to cook fish without the risk of it becoming dry. I make mine by lining the inside of some foil with parchment paper, as I personally don't like to cook directly on foil due to the concerns about aluminum leaching into the food.

Salmon is a source of protein, as well as omega-3 fats. I try to buy sustainably caught wild salmon as I find that the quality of farmed fish can sometimes be harder to judge, although there are now a few more responsible suppliers available if you shop around.

Preheat the oven to 400°F.

Shred the red cabbage. If you are following the meal plan, shred the whole cabbage while you're at it, as you will use the other half to make some Quick Pickled Cabbage (see page 224) later. Prepare the carrots and mix with the cabbage. Then add the cilantro leaves, lime zest, leftover broccoli and sugar snap peas, and mix together well. Split this salad into 2 portions, putting one aside for tomorrow's lunch, a beautiful salmon salad (see page 185).

Next, line a baking tray with foil and lay a sheet of parchment paper on top. Slice the zested lime and lay the slices on the paper. Place the salmon fillets on top, skin down if they have it. Scatter the ginger, scallions, lime zest, and chili on top. Drizzle with a little olive oil, plus a grind of black pepper.

(Recipe continues over page . . .)

FOR THE LIME &
GINGER DRESSING
(makes 2 portions)

2 tablespoons tahini

1 teaspoon tamari or
coconut aminos

1 tablespoon extra-virgin
olive oil

juice of ½ a lime (lemon
works just as well)

½ clove of garlic, peeled
and crushed

¼–½ teaspoon grated
fresh ginger

¼–½ teaspoon honey
or coconut sugar

3 tablespoons cold water

Fold the paper and foil around the fish and ensure it is tightly sealed. Put into the oven and bake for 8–12 minutes (depending on the thickness of your fillet), then remove from the oven, open the parcel a little, and insert a knife into the thickest part of the salmon. If it is opaque, not pink, it is done. If not, reseal the bag and cook for 2–3 minutes more.

While the salmon is cooking, toast the cashews by placing them onto a small tray and roasting for 5 minutes in the oven. Set a timer as they have a tendency to burn.

Whisk or blend all the dressing ingredients together until smooth. Season to taste.

To serve, toss half the salad in 2 tablespoons of the dressing, sprinkle with the toasted cashews, and serve with 1 fillet of salmon on top.

VEGAN ALTERNATIVES

ROASTED VEGETABLES with CASHEW NUT CREAM on TOAST (V)

PYRAMID:

Who says we have to eat sweet carbs for the first meal of the day? I much prefer to enjoy something substantial and savory, like this dish.

1 portion of leftover roasted vegetables

1 slice of gluten-free bread

1 portion of Cashew Nut Cream (see page 159)

a handful of baby leaf salad

a little balsamic vinegar (optional)

Warm up the roasted vegetables gently in a medium oven for 10 minutes or so (although I also like them cold, straight from the fridge!).

Toast the gluten-free bread well, then spread with the Cashew Nut Cream. Top with the vegetables and serve alongside a baby leaf salad, adding a drizzle of balsamic vinegar.

WALNUT LENTIL PÂTÉ (V)

1 tablespoon light olive oil

1 small onion, peeled and roughly chopped

1 clove of garlic, peeled and crushed

3 chestnut mushrooms (about 2 oz), sliced

generous ¾ cup cooked Puy lentils

¼ cup walnuts

2 tablespoons chopped fresh parsley

1 teaspoon chopped fresh sage or basil leaves

2 tablespoons apple cider vinegar

1 tablespoon tahini

2–3 sun-dried tomatoes, drained and chopped

a generous pinch of salt and freshly ground black pepper

TO SERVE

1 Bibb lettuce

a handful of cherry tomatoes

PYRAMID:

This pâté is a great way to use up leftover cooked lentils or other pulses. They're blended with vibrant herbs and sun-dried tomatoes for depth of flavor, with some delicious tahini for creaminess and walnuts for texture. The pâté is great for dipping veggies into, spreading on some gluten-free toast or serving in little lettuce cups as done here.

Heat the olive oil in a small frying pan over low–medium heat. Add the onion, garlic, and sliced mushrooms and sauté for 8–10 minutes, stirring regularly, until softened. Remove from the heat and allow to cool.

Tip this mix together with all the remaining ingredients into a food processor. Pulse until you reach your desired consistency. The pâté should hold its shape when you press a spoonful of the mixture against the side of the bowl. I prefer it a little chunky, but you could keep blending for a smoother consistency if you prefer.

Taste and adjust seasoning as necessary.

If making ahead, place, covered, in the fridge overnight. Spoon into little lettuce cups to serve.

ASIAN-STYLE SALAD (V)

FOR THE SALAD BASE
(makes 2 portions)

½ a small head of red
cabbage, finely sliced

2 small carrots, peeled and
julienned or grated

3 cups leftover steamed
broccoli, sliced

1 cup leftover sugar snap
peas, sliced

zest of 1 lime

½ a bunch of fresh cilantro,
stalks removed, leaves
chopped

FOR THE LIME & GINGER
DRESSING *(see page 172)*

TO SERVE FOR SUPPER

scant ½ cup cashews

½ a red chili pepper, seeded
and finely diced (optional)

PYRAMID:

These beautiful dishes are a fantastic way to bring the rainbow to your plate, and by making one salad base and finishing it two ways, you minimize preparation time while maximizing taste and nutrition. I love Lime & Ginger Dressing too. I'll make a double portion and keep it in the fridge (where it will thicken up and reach an almost mayonnaise-like consistency).

Preheat the oven to 400°F.

Shred the red cabbage. If you are following the meal plan, it might be a good idea to shred the whole cabbage while you're at it, as you will use the other half to make some Quick Pickled Cabbage (see page 224) later.

Prepare the carrots and mix with the cabbage. Then add the leftover broccoli and sugar snap peas, lime zest, and cilantro leaves and mix together well. Split this salad into two portions, putting one aside for tomorrow's lunch.

To make the dressing, whisk all the ingredients together until smooth. You will have enough for two portions (I usually keep it in a little jar in the fridge). Season to taste.

Scatter the cashews onto a baking tray and toast in the oven for 4–5 minutes. Add them to your salad base with the diced chili and toss through half the dressing. Add some extra cilantro leaves to garnish.

COMPLETE TODAY'S PREPARATION

after supper

1. Skim any fat off the chicken stock that may have formed as it cooled. Add a couple of tablespoons into each portion of leftover roast chicken to help keep it moist, and put these into the freezer. Leave the rest of the stock in the fridge.

2. Use the leftover red cabbage from today's supper to make the Quick Pickled Cabbage recipe on page 224.

3. Using the leftover roasted beets, roasted vegetables, and chicken stock from prep day and yesterday, now is a great time to whizz up your soup for Day 5 (see page 206). Once the soup has cooled, it can go in the freezer.

4. When the second portion of salmon has cooled, make up the Salmon Salad in a Jar for tomorrow's lunch (see page 185).

for the vegan plan

1. *Use the leftover red cabbage from today's supper to make the Quick Pickled Cabbage recipe on page 224.*

2. *Using the leftover roasted beets and roasted vegetables, whizz up your soup for Day 5 (see page 210). Once the soup has cooled, this can go in the freezer.*

3. *Prepare your lunch tomorrow (see page 187). It's a good idea to keep the dressing separate from all the salads you prepare ahead of time, only adding it just before eating (or you'll find it goes soggy).*

Mindful Moment

Ask yourself the following question before each meal tomorrow: *How hungry am I on a scale of 1–10?* Learning to interpret "true" hunger from "psychological" hunger (which is often actually boredom or force of habit) is a key skill to master in mindful eating. Here is the hunger scale I use with my clients:

1. LIGHTHEADED AND SHAKY

2. STARVING AND IRRITABLE

3. RUMBLING TUMMY

4. THINKING ABOUT FOOD

5. COULD EAT A LITTLE MORE, BUT GENERALLY OK

6. PERFECTLY SATISFIED

7. A LITTLE FULL

8. LOOSENING THE BELT A NOTCH

9. BLOATED AND UNCOMFORTABLE

10. COMPLETELY STUFFED

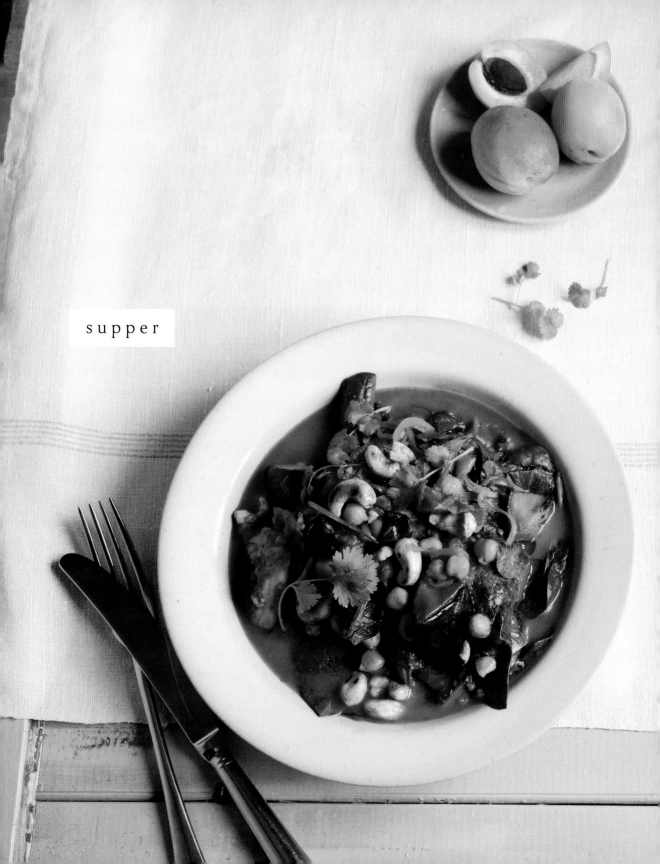

supper

lunch

breakfast

DAY 3

BREAKFAST: BANANA, MINT & LIME SMOOTHIE (v)

LUNCH: SALMON SALAD in a JAR
+ 1 PORTION OF SEASONAL FRUIT

SUPPER: EGGPLANT & CHICKPEA CURRY (v)
+ 1 PORTION of SEASONAL FRUIT

vegan alternative:

LUNCH: ASIAN-STYLE SALAD with MANGO
+ 1 PORTION OF SEASONAL FRUIT

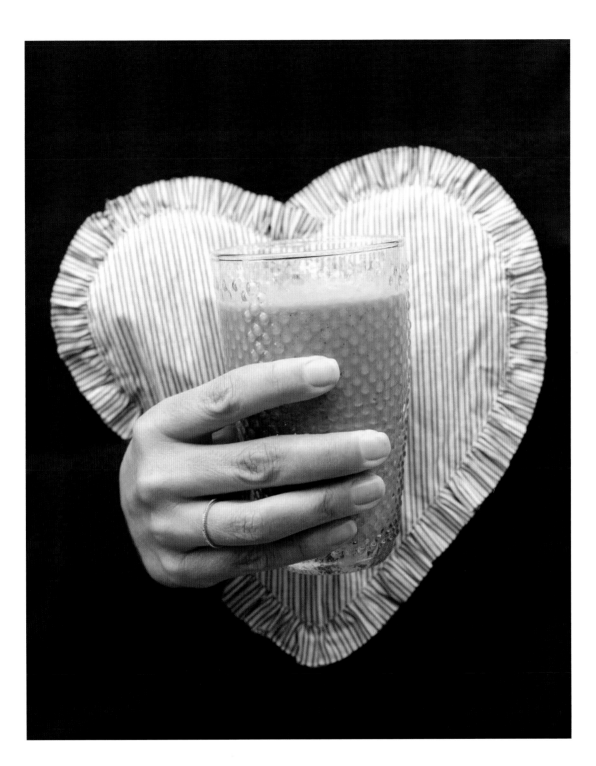

BANANA, MINT & LIME SMOOTHIE (V)

2 tablespoons hulled
hemp seeds, plus
1 teaspoon for the top

½ oz spinach

1 stick of celery,
roughly chopped

2-inch piece of cucumber,
roughly chopped

¼ of an avocado, peeled

½ a large banana, peeled
and frozen if possible

10 mint leaves, plus a couple
for the top to garnish

zest and juice of 1 lime

¾ cup coconut water or
cold water

PYRAMID:

A smoothie can be a good breakfast option for busy days. This green one is both tasty and filling, with protein from the hemp seeds and healthy fats from the avocado. I tend to freeze bananas that are starting to go a little overripe, and these work particularly well in this recipe.

Combine all the ingredients in a blender and whizz until smooth, adding a little more coconut water or cold water if necessary to reach the desired consistency.

Pour over ice if you want, and top with a teaspoon of hemp seeds before serving.

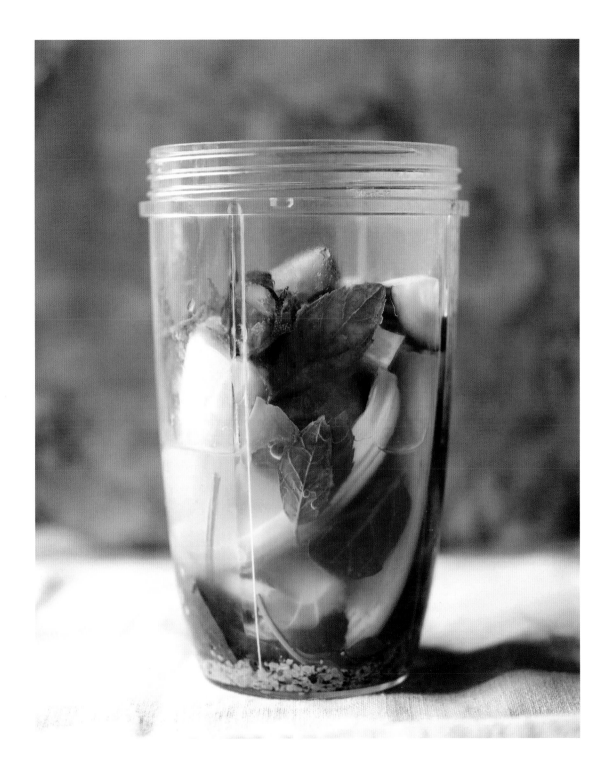

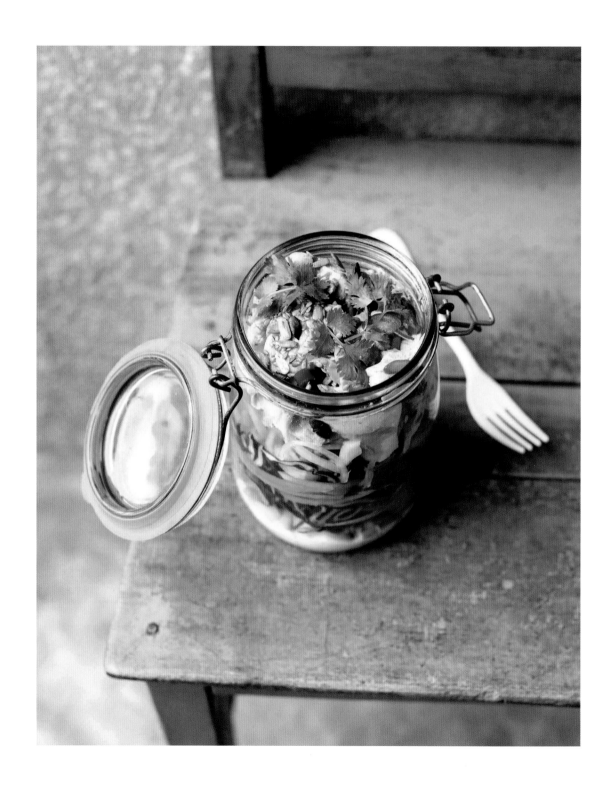

SALMON SALAD in a JAR

PYRAMID:

This salad is so easy and versatile. It would be just as delicious with chicken or shrimp instead. I find packing salads in jars helps to stop the vegetables going soggy (make sure you put the dressing in the bottom, though), and it's a very convenient way to transport food if you are on the move. The ultimate packed lunch.

2 tablespoons Lime & Ginger Dressing (see page 172)

¼ of an avocado, peeled and cubed

a drizzle of lime juice

1 portion of leftover Asian-style Salad (see page 171)

4–5 cherry tomatoes, cut into quarters

½ a cucumber, spiralized

1 salmon fillet, cooked and flaked

a few cilantro leaves (optional)

1 teaspoon fresh chili pepper, finely diced (or dried chili flakes)

2 tablespoons Spiced Seed Sprinkle (see page 140)

2 lime wedges, to serve

Put the dressing in the bottom of a large Mason jar or jam jar.

Add the avocado cubes (with a drizzle of lime juice), followed by the leftover salad. Put the tomatoes in next, then add the spiralized cucumber on top. Lastly, add your flaked salmon fillet.

Add a few cilantro leaves if you like, then a sprinkle of chili and the toasted seed mix. Finally, put the lime wedges on top, ready to squeeze over when you eat the salad.

If making ahead, it will keep well in the fridge overnight.

EGGPLANT & CHICKPEA CURRY (V)

MAKES: 2 portions

2 tablespoons coconut oil or light olive oil

1 onion, peeled and sliced

1-inch piece of fresh ginger, peeled

3 cloves of garlic, peeled

½ teaspoon turmeric

½ teaspoon chili powder

1 teaspoon ground cumin

2 teaspoons ground coriander

1 teaspoon garam masala

½ teaspoon salt

6 ripe tomatoes, chopped

2½ cups vegetable stock (or chicken stock for non-vegans, see page 156)

½ an eggplant, cubed

generous ⅓ cup cashew nuts

1 x 14 oz can of chickpeas, drained and well rinsed

a bunch of fresh finely chopped cilantro

2 handfuls of spinach

freshly ground black pepper

juice of 1 lime

TO SERVE FOR LUNCH TOMORROW

a handful of seasonal greens

PYRAMID:

If you're anything like me, this curry may well become a firm favorite in your recipe repertoire as soon as you've taken the first bite. It's a bowl of pure, wholesome, warming goodness. It really is worth using fresh tomatoes if you can find ripe ones.

In a heavy-bottomed pot, heat the oil over medium heat, then add the onion and cook to soften. Grate the ginger and chop the garlic. Turn down the heat to low, then stir in the ginger and garlic into the onion and cook for another minute or so. Add the dry spices and salt, and cook for a further 30 seconds. Add the chopped tomatoes and the stock, then cook for 10 minutes, uncovered, stirring regularly to break down the tomatoes with the back of the spoon.

Once the tomatoes have cooked down and reduced a little to make a sauce, add the eggplant cubes, cashews, and chickpeas. Stir well to coat them with the tomatoes, then cover and cook again, still over low heat, for another 10–12 minutes until soft. You may need to add some water if it looks a little too thick. Stir occasionally to stop it sticking to the bottom.

Finally, add the cilantro and spinach leaves, and cook for a couple of minutes, until they have wilted. Taste and check for seasoning.

Serve half the curry topped with half the cilantro and a squeeze of lime juice. Leave the other half to cool before refrigerating. Serve for lunch tomorrow with your seasonal greens.

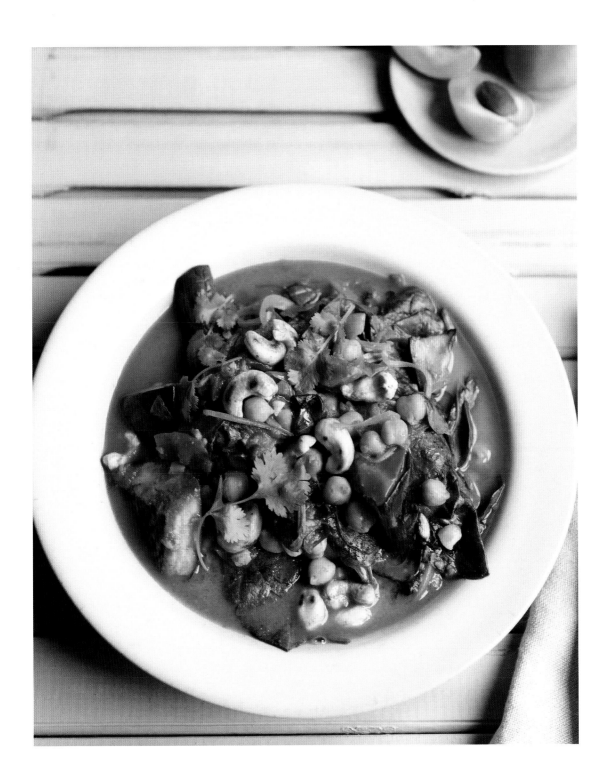

VEGAN ALTERNATIVE

ASIAN-STYLE SALAD with MANGO (V)

¾ cup chopped mango

½ a red chili pepper, seeded and finely diced (optional)

juice of ½ a lime

1 portion leftover Asian-style Salad (see page 175)

a portion of Lime & Ginger Dressing (see page 172)

3 tablespoons Spiced Seed Sprinkle (see page 140)

PYRAMID:

Add the chopped mango, chili and lime juice to the Asian-style salad base. If you're preparing this the day before, keep it in an airtight container in the fridge overnight.

Toss through the dressing and add the toasted seeds just before serving.

COMPLETE TODAY'S PREPARATION

after supper

for both the main plan and the vegan plan

1. Soak oats for the Overnight Oat Crumble (see page 196) for breakfast tomorrow morning.

2. Once the second portion of Eggplant & Chickpea Curry has cooled, transfer to a container, add a generous handful of your choice of greens, and leave it covered in the fridge ready for lunch tomorrow.

Mindful Moment

Turn off all screens and shut all books, papers, or magazines before eating your meals tomorrow. Eating while distracted reduces our focus on the food in front of us. The more we focus on our meals with *all* of our senses, the more satisfied we can feel at the end of them.

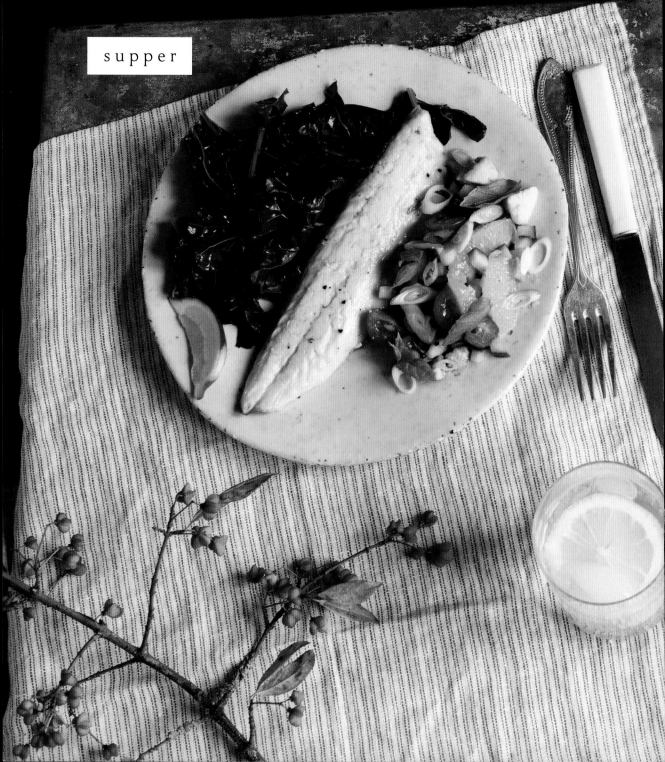

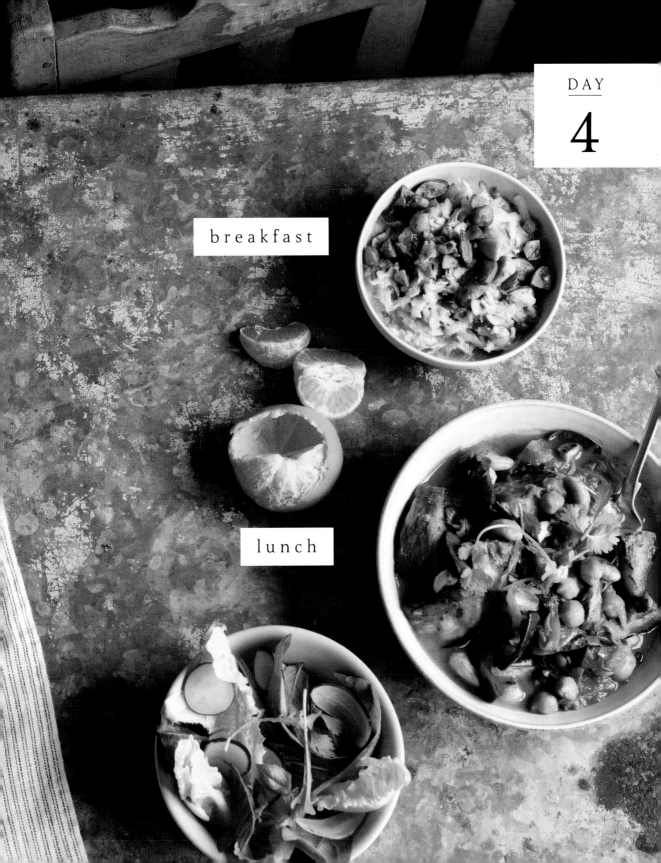

DAY
4

breakfast

lunch

DAY 4

BREAKFAST: OVERNIGHT OAT CRUMBLE with APPLE (v)

LUNCH: LEFTOVER EGGPLANT & CHICKPEA CURRY (see page 186) (v)
+ 1 PORTION of SEASONAL FRUIT

SUPPER: GRILLED FISH with ORANGE & AVOCADO SALSA

vegan alternatives:

SUPPER: SMOKED TOFU with ORANGE &
AVOCADO SALSA

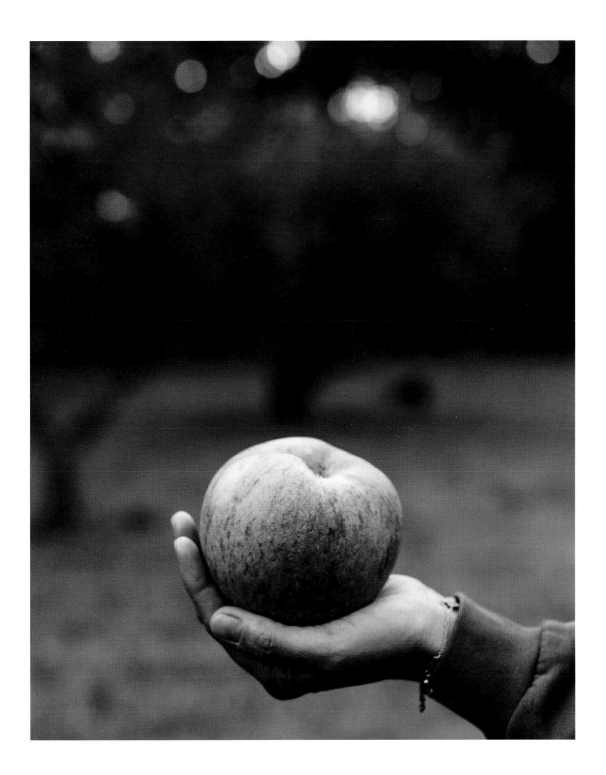

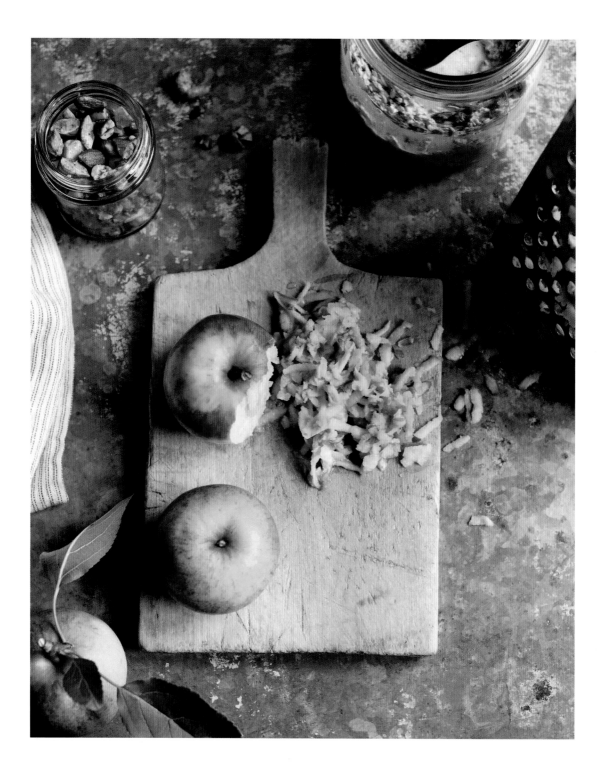

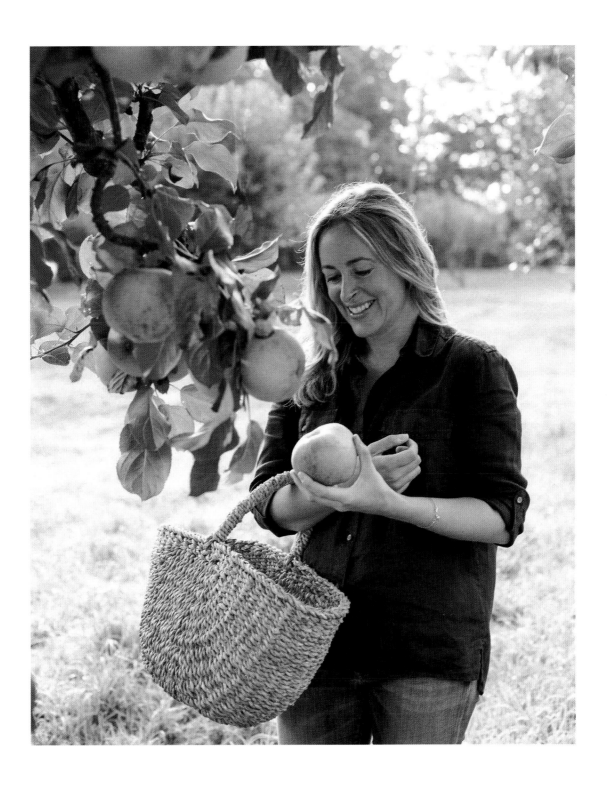

OVERNIGHT OAT CRUMBLE (V)

MAKES: *2 portions*

¾ cup almond or unsweetened coconut milk (from a carton)

¾ cup gluten-free oats

1 teaspoon ground cinnamon

TO SERVE FOR BREAKFAST ON DAY 4

1 apple, grated (although leave the skin on for the extra fiber and phytonutrients)

2 tablespoons sultanas

3 tablespoons Nut Granola (see page 141)

TO SERVE FOR BREAKFAST ON DAY 5

1 cup fresh berries (I love to use blackberries when they are in season, but any berry works well)

3 tablespoons Nut Granola (see page 141)

PYRAMID:

Overnight oats are very easy and quick to make in advance, so they are great for an early start or when traveling.

I have served this breakfast in two slightly different ways for variety. However, you will use the same soaked base mix to make both, so it only takes a minute to throw together in the morning.

Oats can boost the nutritional value of a gluten-free diet, by adding an extra source of B vitamins, zinc, and magnesium. Plus the fiber in oats, called beta-glucan, not only helps you to feel fuller for longer but has also been found to reduce the levels of some hunger hormones.

Mix the milk, oats, and ground cinnamon together and divide between two covered bowls (or even better, two jars with lids). Leave in the fridge overnight to soak. They will keep for 2–3 days like this.

In the morning, add the suggested toppings to the soaked oats before serving.

VARIATIONS Overnight oats are the ideal recipe to play around with according to the seasons. Just use the basic overnight oat mix (the milk and oats, opposite), then try adding the following for flavor, or make up your own new favorite.

- Add a handful of fresh blueberries, raspberries, and a few almonds to the oats before soaking overnight for a berry burst.

- Add a mashed ripe banana or ½ cup to ¾ cup of diced mango and a spoonful of coconut chips to your oats before soaking, for a sweet, tropical flavor.

- Mix in a teaspoon or two of organic cocoa powder and a little sweetener (such as honey) for a chocolate hit. You could add a handful of toasted hazelnuts too instead of the Nut Granola.

- Layer up a homemade seasonal fruit compote (try rhubarb in spring, strawberry in summer, and blackberry or apple in autumn) with your oat mix before serving. Just put a spoonful of compote into a glass, top with a spoonful of soaked oats, then another spoonful of compote and keep going until you have a beautiful fruity-oat sundae!

GRILLED FISH with ORANGE & AVOCADO SALSA

1 fillet of sea bass or another seasonal white fish (if you are using frozen fillets, allow them to defrost thoroughly before cooking)

1 tablespoon olive oil

a wedge of lime

freshly ground black pepper

FOR THE SALSA

¼ of an avocado, peeled and diced

zest of ½ a lime

a pinch of sea salt

1 scallion, sliced

4-inch piece of cucumber, seeded and diced

6–8 cherry tomatoes, cut into quarters

1 orange, peeled and segmented

2 tablespoons chopped fresh mint leaves

TO SERVE

1–2 handfuls of salad leaves (arugula works well) or steamed greens

PYRAMID:

I first tried this zingy salsa when I was working in Sicily many years ago and although I have changed it along the way (it originally had grapefruit in it), it is now a firm favorite and works brilliantly alongside a simple grilled fillet of fish or some shrimp. The orange gives a really fresh touch with the avocado and mint. White fish provides an important source of dietary iodine, which is essential for normal thyroid function.

Preheat the broiler to 425°F or its highest setting. Place an oven rack near the top of the oven, and lightly oil a baking tray.

While the broiler is heating up, mix all the salsa ingredients together in a bowl and taste for seasoning.

Lay the fish skin side up on your prepared baking tray. Make three or four cuts in the skin at the thickest part of the fillet (if it has no skin you won't need to do this). Drizzle with olive oil, squeeze over a little lime juice, and add a grind of black pepper.

Cook for 4–5 minutes under the hot broiler until the flesh is cooked. This will take slightly longer if you have a thicker fish, such as halibut or cod. Insert a knife into the thickest part of the fish and if it is not yet opaque, it needs a little longer.

Serve on a bed of salad leaves or steamed greens, with the salsa alongside.

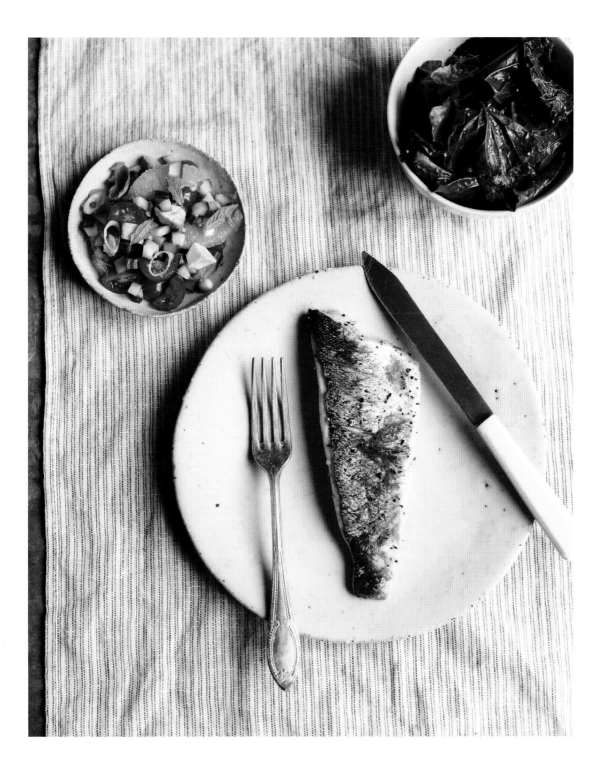

VEGAN ALTERNATIVE

SMOKED TOFU with ORANGE & AVOCADO SALSA (V)

4 oz smoked tofu

1 tablespoon extra-virgin olive oil

a wedge of lime

freshly ground black pepper

FOR THE SALSA

¼ of an avocado, peeled and diced

zest of ½ a lime

a pinch of sea salt

1 scallion, sliced

4-inch piece of cucumber, seeded and diced

6–8 cherry tomatoes, cut into quarters

1 orange, peeled and segmented

2 tablespoons chopped fresh mint leaves

TO SERVE

1–2 handfuls of salad leaves (arugula works well) or steamed winter greens

PYRAMID: **2 1 1 3**

This generous portion of salsa is a lovely salad on its own, but is also a great accompaniment to all sorts of dishes. Although I don't advocate eating too much smoked food, it is OK once in a while, and works particularly well here.

Preheat your broiler to 425°F or its highest setting.

Place a rack near the top of the oven, and lightly oil a baking tray.

While the broiler is heating up, mix all the salsa ingredients together in a bowl and taste for seasoning.

Lay the tofu on the baking tray. Drizzle with olive oil, squeeze over lime juice, and add a grind of black pepper.

Cook for 4–5 minutes under the hot broiler, then flip over and grill for another 4 minutes on the other side, or until hot through and golden.

Serve on a bed of salad leaves or steamed greens, with the salsa alongside.

COMPLETE TODAY'S PREPARATION

after supper

1. Take the Roasted Vegetable & Chicken Soup out of the freezer, along with a portion of your pre-cooked roast chicken, so that they are defrosted in time for lunch tomorrow

for the vegan plan

1. *Take the Roasted Vegetable Soup out of the freezer to defrost in time for lunch tomorrow.*

Mindful Moment

Try eating with your non-dominant hand for at least one of your meals tomorrow. Swapping your knife and fork over breaks an ingrained habit, and by doing so, activates your brain into concentrating a little more on the action of eating.

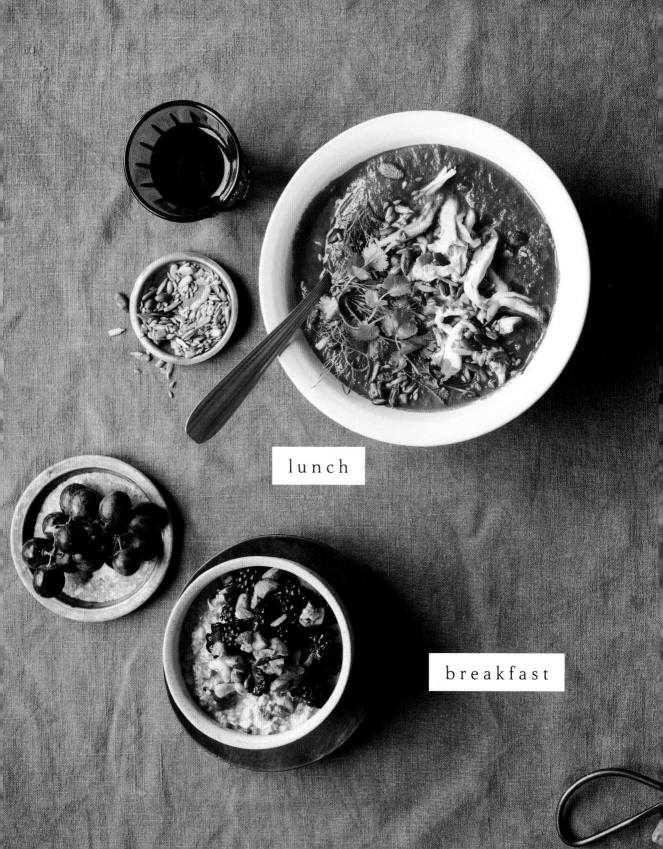

lunch

breakfast

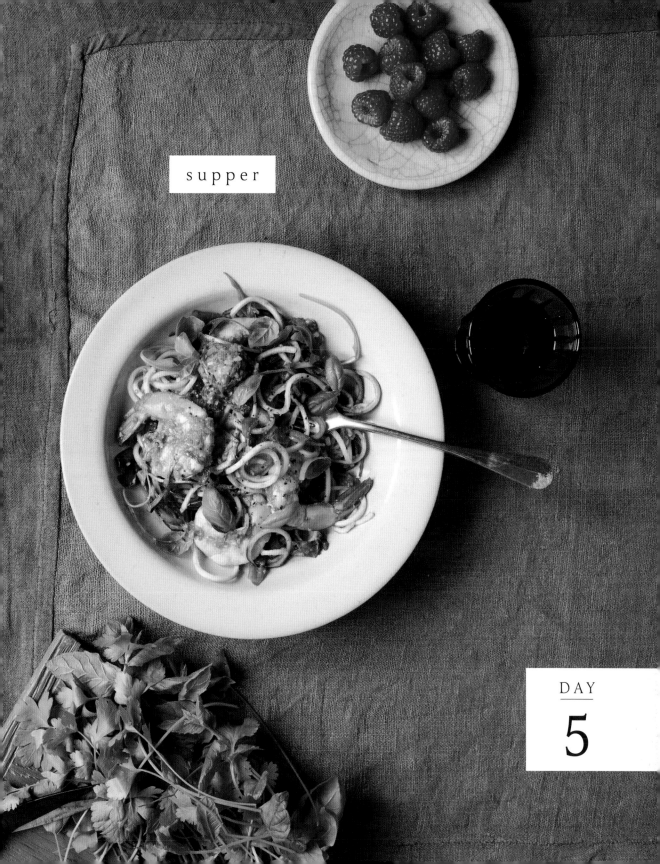

supper

DAY 5

BREAKFAST: OVERNIGHT OAT CRUMBLE with BERRIES
(see page 196) (v)

LUNCH: ROASTED VEGETABLE & CHICKEN SOUP
+ 1 PORTION of SEASONAL FRUIT

SUPPER: SPICY TOMATO & SHRIMP ZUCCHINI NOODLES
+ 1 PORTION of SEASONAL FRUIT

---

vegan alternatives:

LUNCH: ROASTED VEGETABLE SOUP
+ 1 PORTION of SEASONAL FRUIT

SUPPER: SPICY TOMATO & LIMA BEAN ZUCCHINI NOODLES
+ 1 PORTION of SEASONAL FRUIT

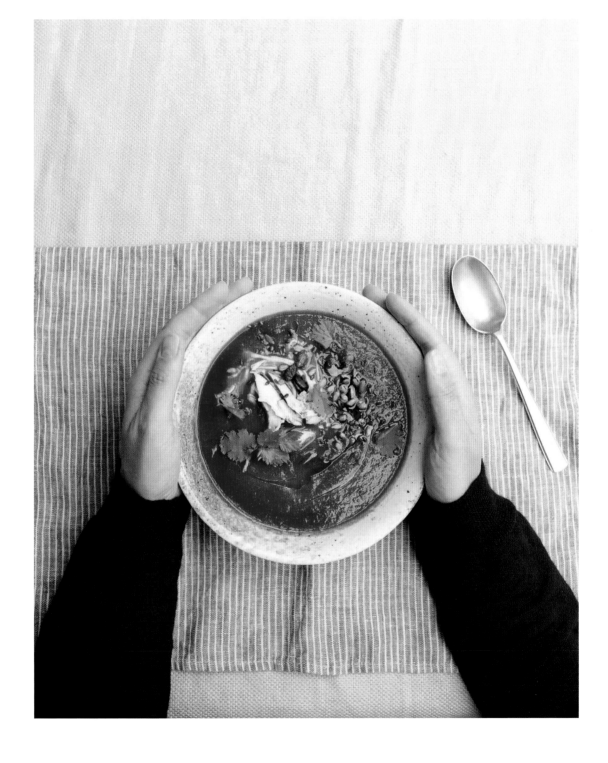

ROASTED VEGETABLE & CHICKEN SOUP

PYRAMID:

The nutritional benefits of beets have been linked to all sorts of health benefits, from improved blood flow and athletic stamina to reductions in blood pressure. I also think they are super delicious, and this soup of leftovers is one of my favorite ways to enjoy them.

1 portion of leftover roasted vegetables

1 portion of leftover roasted beets, peeled and roughly chopped (about 1–2 medium beets)

2½ cups homemade Chicken Stock (see page 156)

sea salt and freshly ground black pepper, to taste

TO SERVE

1 portion (about 5 oz) of leftover roast chicken, chopped

a small handful of fresh herbs of your choice, roughly chopped

2–3 tablespoons Spiced Seed Sprinkle (see page 140)

a drizzle of extra-virgin olive oil

Place the leftover roasted vegetables, peeled beets, and chicken stock into a pot and bring to a simmer for 5 minutes or so.

Turn off the heat and blend thoroughly. Taste and season. If you are making it ahead of time, allow it to cool completely before freezing.

Before serving, reheat the soup and the chicken pieces thoroughly (I do this separately, but you could also just mix it all in together). Serve in a bowl, topped with fresh herbs, toasted seeds, and a drizzle of extra-virgin olive oil.

Please note, this makes a very generous portion of soup, so don't worry if you can't finish it all! Just eat until you are satisfied.

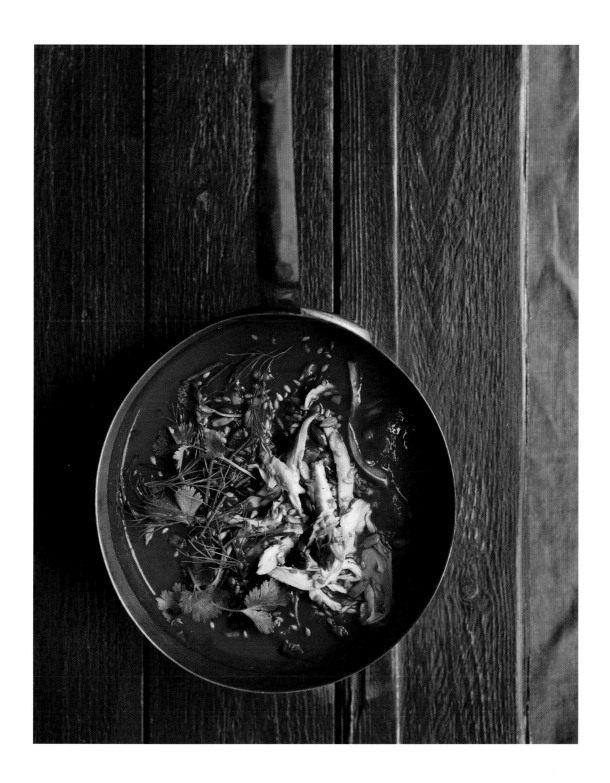

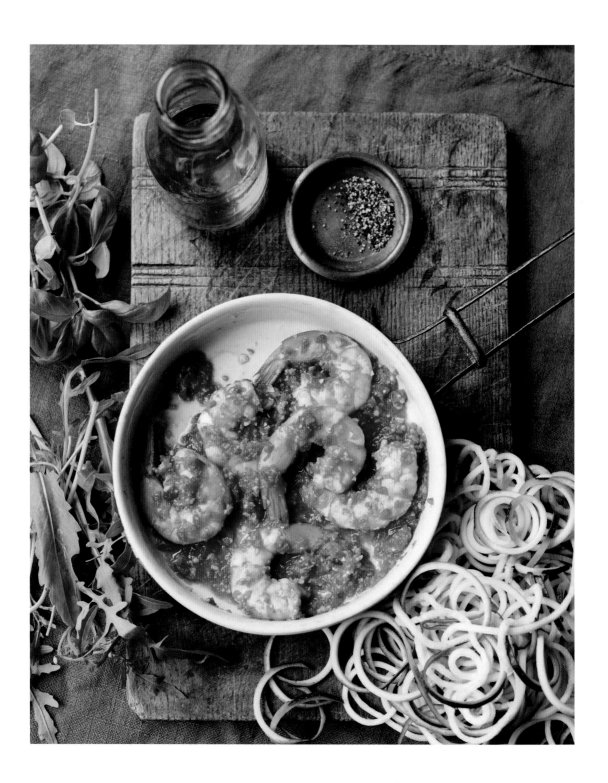

SPICY TOMATO & SHRIMP ZUCCHINI NOODLES

PYRAMID:

I have been making this dish for years and just love it. It's a rich and tasty bowl of goodness, just as satisfying as eating any bowl of pasta. And it takes only a few minutes to make. Tomatoes contain all sorts of health-giving compounds, including lycopene, and powerful antioxidants such as vitamins E and C. Eating tomatoes alongside olive oil can actually boost your absorption of some of these beneficial compounds, so it seems like the Italians have it exactly right!

8–10 cherry tomatoes

1 clove of garlic, peeled

1 red chili pepper (remove the seeds if you don't like it too spicy), chopped

1–2 tablespoons tomato puree

sea salt and freshly ground black pepper, to taste

1 tablespoon light olive oil

4½ oz jumbo shrimp, no shells (defrosted if using frozen shrimp)

a large handful of arugula

1 zucchini, spiralized or grated

a bunch of finely chopped fresh basil or flat-leaved parsley

a drizzle of extra-virgin olive oil

lemon zest (optional)

Put the cherry tomatoes, garlic, chopped chili, tomato puree, a pinch of salt, and some black pepper into a small blender (I use my handheld blender, which has a jug attachment). Blend to a sauce consistency.

Heat the oil in a wide saucepan, then add the spicy tomato sauce from the blender and simmer for a few minutes. You may need to add a little water if it's on the thick side.

Add the shrimp and simmer for a further 4–5 minutes, or until they are cooked through. Add the arugula and stir through to wilt.

Toss the zucchini noodles through the mix, just until it begins to soften. Sprinkle with the fresh herbs, a little extra-virgin olive oil, lemon zest, and season to taste. Serve immediately.

ROASTED VEGETABLE SOUP (V)

1 portion of leftover
roasted vegetables

1 portion of leftover
roasted beets, peeled
and roughly chopped (about
1–2 medium beets)

2¼ cups vegetable stock

sea salt and freshly ground
black pepper, to taste

TO SERVE

2 tablespoons dairy-free
coconut yogurt (optional)

a small handful of
fresh herbs of your choice,
roughly chopped

3 tablespoons Spiced Seed
Sprinkle (see page 140)

1–2 handfuls of salad leaves
(arugula and spinach go well
with this soup)

a drizzle of extra-virgin
olive oil

a wedge of lemon

PYRAMID:

This deep purple-red soup is not only beautiful but tastes wonderful too. Adding in some toasted seeds and a lovely green salad, dressed with olive oil and lemon juice, makes a very filling and nutritious meal.

Place the leftover roasted vegetables, beets, and stock into a pot and bring to a simmer for 5 minutes or so.

Turn off the heat and blend thoroughly. Taste and season. If you are making this ahead of time, allow it to cool completely at this point, before freezing.

Before serving, reheat the soup well. Serve topped with a dollop of coconut yogurt, some fresh herbs, and a sprinkle of seeds.

Dress the salad leaves with a generous drizzle of olive oil and lemon juice and serve alongside.

SPICY TOMATO &
LIMA BEAN ZUCCHINI NOODLES (V)

8–10 cherry tomatoes

1 scallion,
roughly chopped

1 clove of garlic, peeled

1 red chili pepper

1–2 tablespoons
tomato puree

1 tablespoon olive oil

1 cup lima beans, chopped

2–3 sun-dried tomatoes,
drained and chopped

a large handful of arugula

1 zucchini, spiralized

FOR THE PESTO

2 tablespoons olive oil

juice of ½ a lemon

2 tablespoons chopped
fresh basil leaves

2 tablespoons fresh
parsley leaves

1 tablespoon pine nuts
(or sunflower seeds)

a good pinch of sea salt and
freshly ground black pepper

TO SERVE

a few leaves of fresh basil,
to garnish

1 tablespoon pine nuts

PYRAMID:

Sometimes I just feel like a hearty bowl of something simple, and this dish fits the bill perfectly. Rustled up from ingredients you're likely to have lying around (you can always substitute a different type of bean for the lima beans if you want), this is a nutritious meal that can be on the table in minutes.

In a small blender (I use my handheld blender with a jug attachment), mix the cherry tomatoes, scallion, garlic, chili, and tomato puree with a pinch of salt and blend to a sauce consistency.

Heat the oil in a wide saucepan, then add the spicy tomato sauce from the blender and simmer for a few minutes. You may need to add a little water if it's on the thick side.

While this is simmering, rinse out the blender jug you've just used. Combine all the pesto ingredients in the jug and blend for a minute or so, until well combined. If it looks a little dry, you can always add an extra squeeze of lemon juice. Taste and season accordingly.

Add the lima beans and the sun-dried tomatoes to the tomato sauce and simmer for 4–5 minutes, until they are heated through. Then add the arugula and stir through to wilt. Remove from the heat.

Toss the zucchini noodles through the warm tomato mix, just until it begins to soften. Serve drizzled with a tablespoon of the fresh pesto, some extra basil leaves, and the rest of the pine nuts. Refrigerate the leftover pesto for later in the plan.

COMPLETE TODAY'S PREPARATION

after supper

1. Prepare the Smoked Salmon & Kale Waldorf salad for lunch tomorrow (see page 220).

2. Peel and chop a ripe banana and put it into the freezer for the Nutty Banana Nice Cream tomorrow night (see page 227).

for the vegan plan

1. *Prepare the Kale Waldorf Salad for lunch tomorrow (see page 228).*

2. *Peel and chop a ripe banana and put it into the freezer for the Nutty Banana Nice Cream tomorrow night (see page 227).*

Mindful Moment

Before one of your meals tomorrow, take a whole minute (set a timer if necessary) to fully appreciate your food before starting to eat. What does it *look* like? What does it *smell* like? *Who* was involved in bringing it to your plate (the farmers, producers, shopkeepers, and cook)? Take a moment to feel gratitude for the blessing of nutritious food.

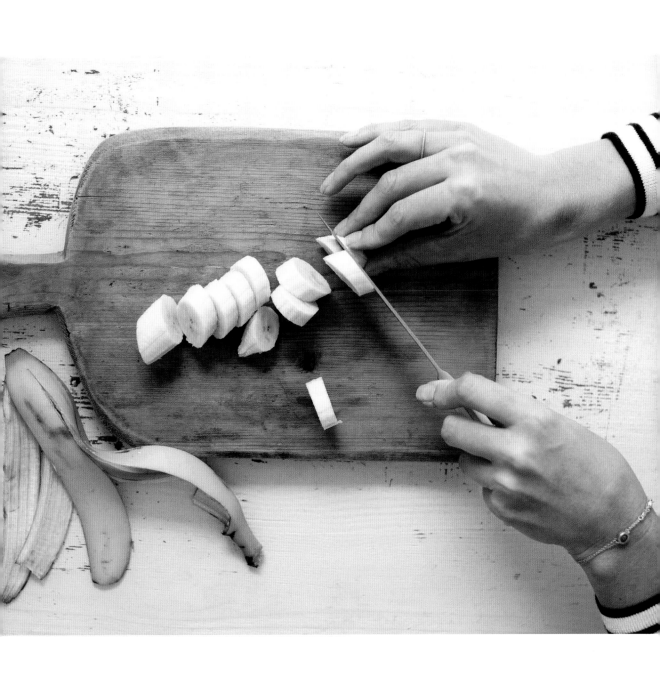

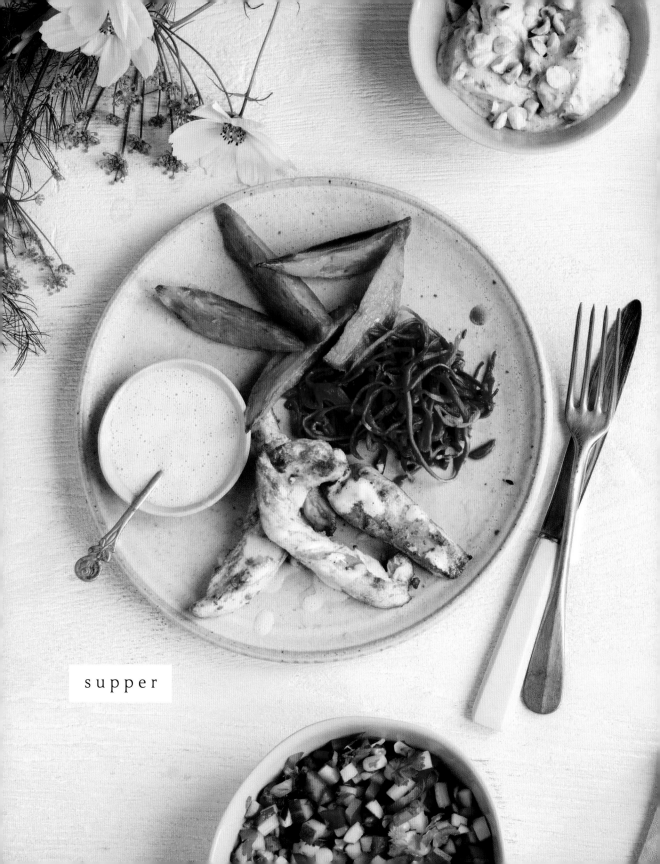

supper

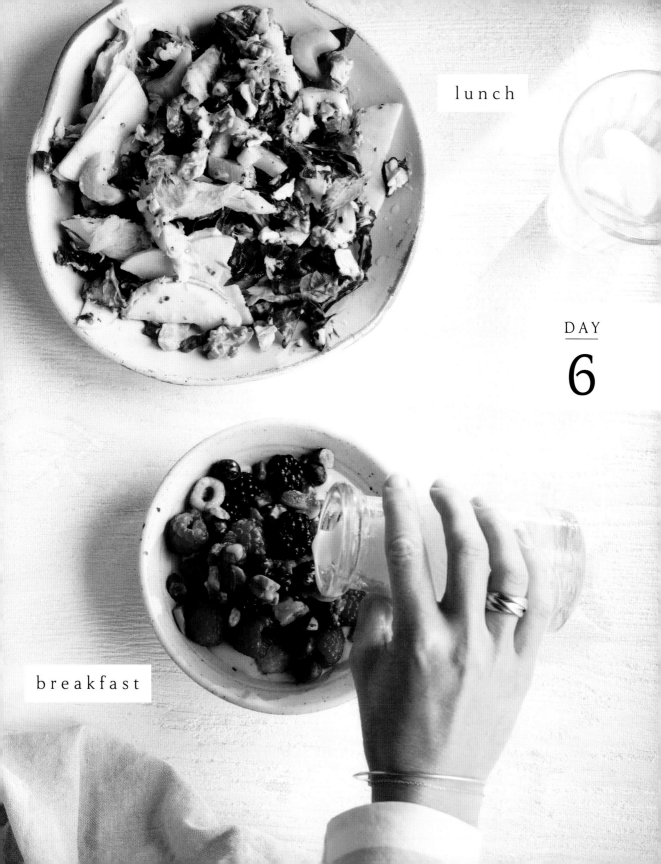

lunch

DAY

6

breakfast

DAY 6

BREAKFAST: NUT GRANOLA with BERRIES (v)

LUNCH: SMOKED SALMON & KALE WALDORF SALAD

SUPPER: CHICKEN & CHIPS with CHOPPED SALAD
+ NUTTY BANANA NICE CREAM

---

vegan alternatives:

LUNCH: KALE WALDORF SALAD

SUPPER: CHOPPED SALAD with SWEET POTATO FRIES
+ NUTTY BANANA NICE CREAM

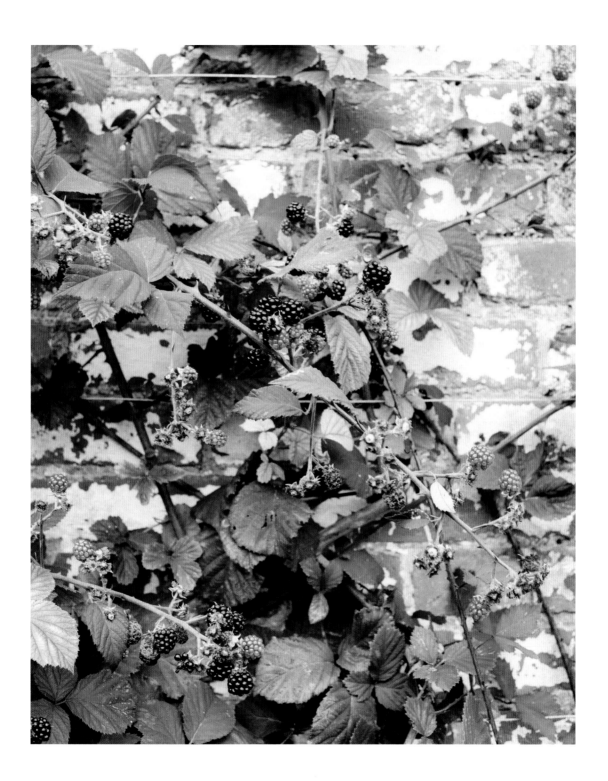

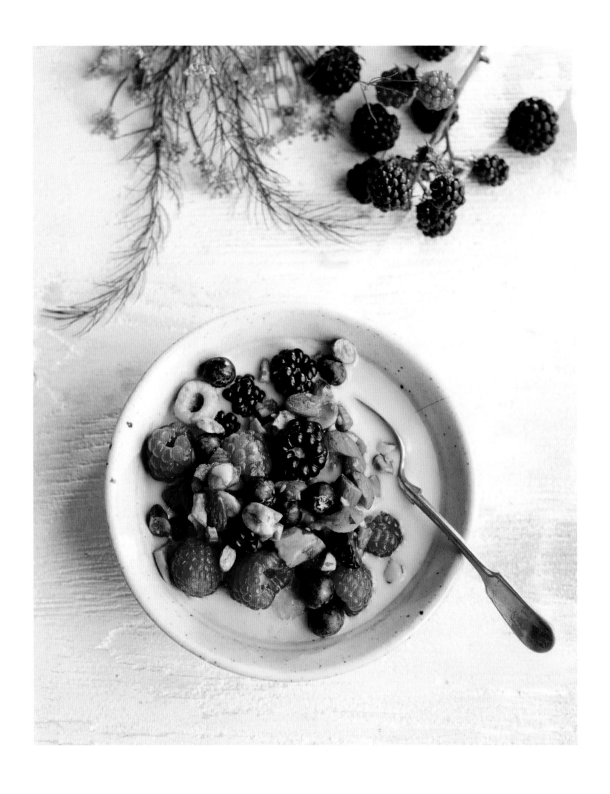

NUT GRANOLA with BERRIES (V)

PYRAMID:

Berries are a tasty and nutritious addition to any diet, potentially supporting heart and gut health, working as potent antioxidants, reducing inflammation, and even helping to stabilize blood sugars. If you are doing this program in winter, you can use frozen berries instead of fresh—just defrost them first.

3 tablespoons Nut Granola
(see page 141)

1 cup fresh berries

½ cup unsweetened coconut milk (from a carton) or almond milk

Alternatively, you may prefer to serve your granola and berries with a big dollop of coconut yogurt (this is dairy-free yogurt made from coconuts, not a coconut-flavored dairy yogurt, just to be clear)

This doesn't really need a recipe, simply mix everything in a bowl and enjoy!

SMOKED SALMON & KALE WALDORF SALAD

1 apple, cored and sliced

juice of ½ a lemon

3½ oz wild or organic smoked salmon, skin removed and broken into pieces

1 stick of celery, sliced

2 handfuls of kale, spinach, or other seasonal leafy greens, woody stems removed and finely sliced

scant ⅓ cup walnuts (1 small handful), roughly chopped

FOR THE DRESSING

2 tablespoons dairy-free coconut yogurt (or 1 tablespoon full-fat organic mayonnaise)

zest and juice of ½ a lemon

1 teaspoon whole-grain mustard

a pinch of sea salt and freshly ground black pepper, to taste

1 tablespoon extra-virgin olive oil

a few leaves of fresh tarragon, finely sliced (optional, but does add a lovely layer of flavor)

PYRAMID:

This simple salad is filling, without leaving you feeling stuffed and sleepy for the rest of the afternoon. It really benefits from being made the night before, so the leaves can soften and the flavors meld together. Just keep the walnuts separate or they may turn a little bitter.

———————————

Toss the apple slices in a bowl with the lemon juice so they don't brown, then remove, and mix with the salmon, celery, and greens.

Whisk the dressing ingredients together. If you are using kale, dress the salad the night before.

If you are making the salad on the day, however, you may prefer to use a more tender leaf, such as spinach, instead.

Add the chopped walnuts just before serving.

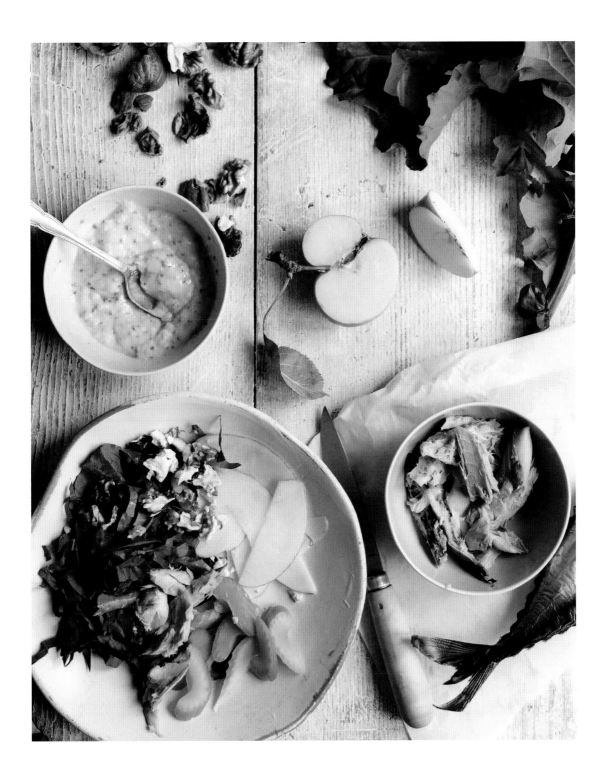

CHICKEN & CHIPS with CHOPPED SALAD

FOR THE CHICKEN AND
CHIPS (*makes 2 portions*)

11 oz sweet potatoes, washed

1 tablespoon light olive oil

1 teaspoon ground cumin

1 teaspoon ground coriander

2 chicken breasts, cut
into strips

FOR THE CHOPPED SALAD
(*makes 2 portions*)

1 red pepper, seeds removed
and diced

heaping ½ cup sweet corn

1 stick of celery, finely diced

2 ripe medium tomatoes,
finely diced

4-inch piece of cucumber,
seeded and finely diced

5–6 radishes, finely diced
(optional)

3–4 tablespoons chopped
fresh parsley or other fresh
herbs (optional)

TO SERVE

2 tablespoons Quick Pickled
Cabbage (see page 225)

2 tablespoons Tahini
Dressing (see page 224)

PYRAMID: 4

This original take on the classically British weekend staple of chicken and chips is delicious! It is absolutely my kind of comfort food. With a wonderfully vibrant salad and tahini dressing alongside, who says tasty treats can't also be healthy?

Preheat the oven to 400°F.

Chop half the sweet potatoes into wedges. Coat with the olive oil and half the ground spices, and season well. Spread out on one half of a baking tray.

Peel the remaining sweet potatoes. Chop into chunks, coat with olive oil (but no need for the spices on these), and spread on the other half of the baking tray. These will be used to make a fritter for breakfast tomorrow.

Put into the oven for 30–35 minutes, or until cooked through and starting to brown around the edges.

Meanwhile, sauté the chicken strips in a frying pan with a little oil and the other half of the ground spices until cooked all the way through.

Finally, mix together all the ingredients for the chopped salad. Season with salt and pepper.

Serve the sweet potato fries, half the cooked chicken, and half of the salad for supper tonight, with the dressing and some tangy pickled cabbage on the side.

Place the peeled sweet potato chunks in a bowl to cool down for breakfast tomorrow.

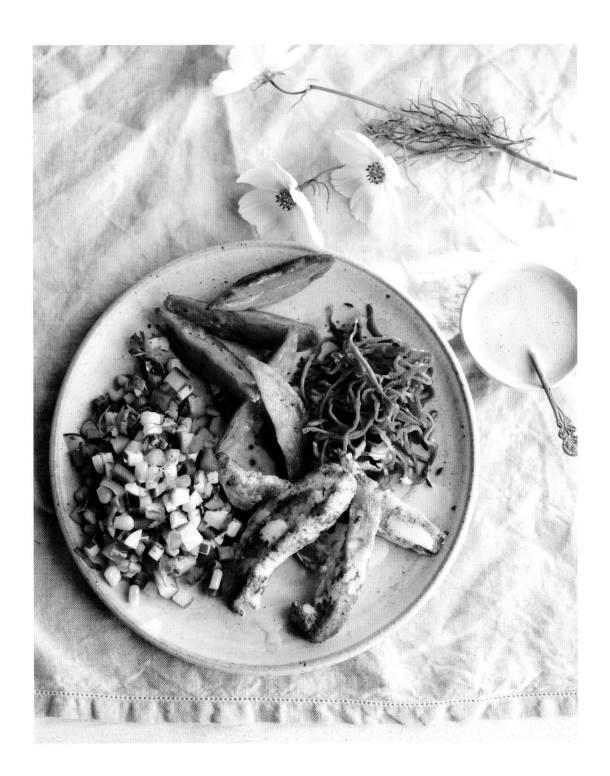

QUICK PICKLED CABBAGE (V)

PYRAMID:

This is my cheater's version of sauerkraut, though "real" sauerkraut is probably better for you because of the fermentation process, which produces lots of gut-friendly bacteria. Give it a try if you have time (there is a full recipe on my website, ameliafreer.com). This recipe is still a great way to add some extra color to your plate, along with some zingy flavors. It's easy and quick (of course!) and keeps for a week in the fridge. You could experiment by changing the type of cabbage and the flavors you add.

¼ cup plus 1 tablespoon water

4 tablespoons apple cider vinegar

1 teaspoon sea salt flakes

1 tablespoon sweetener of choice (such as honey or maple syrup)

1 clove of garlic, peeled and lightly crushed but kept in one piece

1 teaspoon caraway seeds (optional)

½ a small red cabbage, finely sliced

Mix the water, vinegar, salt, and sweetener until dissolved. Add the garlic, caraway seeds, and cabbage and stir well, then put into an airtight container.

Leave to stand for roughly 24 hours at room temperature. This tastes better after a day of pickling, and the flavor will continue to mature. Then store in the fridge for up to a week, stirring and shaking every few days. The cabbage will reduce in volume and the mixture will become more wet, which is to be expected.

Use 2–3 tablespoons per serving.

TAHINI DRESSING (V)

MAKES: 4 portions

PYRAMID: 1

I have been making versions of this dressing for a good few years. It will bring the dullest of dishes to life, and is great to have in your fridge. Sesame seeds (which make tahini) provide a wide array of nutrients such as calcium, iron, magnesium, and zinc, and are a rich source of heart-healthy fats. So this is definitely a good-for-you dressing!

4 tablespoons tahini

2 teaspoons tamari or coconut aminos

2 tablespoons extra-virgin olive oil

¼–½ cup cold water

1 clove of garlic, peeled and crushed

a pinch of sea salt (optional)

juice of 1 lime (½ a lemon works just as well)

Using a small whisk or a blender, combine all the ingredients, apart from the lime or lemon juice, until smooth. Then add the lime or lemon juice. Check the consistency and add more water if it is too thick for your liking. Season to taste.

Store in an airtight container in the fridge for 4–5 days. I tend to use an old, clean jam jar. It will thicken slightly as it cools.

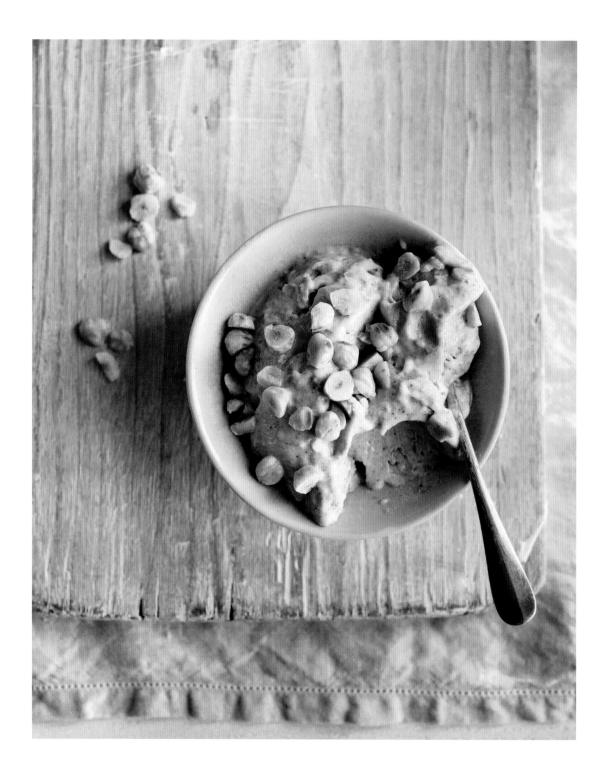

NUTTY BANANA NICE CREAM (V)

1 ripe banana, peeled,
sliced, and frozen

2 teaspoons almond
or hazelnut butter

3 tablespoons coconut or
almond milk

PYRAMID:

If you are not yet familiar with using bananas to make "ice cream," you are in for a real treat. Their texture once frozen and blended is like the most delicious, creamy, sweet ice cream you've ever tasted. The addition of nut butter here adds some healthy fats and plant protein, to slow down the release of fruit sugars from the banana.

Slice and freeze your banana the night before you make this.

In a small food processor or blender, whizz up the banana and nut butter with 2 tablespoons of milk. Push the mixture down the sides of the bowl and add another tablespoon of the milk. Use just enough to get it whizzed up smoothly without becoming runny.

Eat immediately, as it defrosts quickly (although I'm sure I won't need to tell you twice!).

VEGAN ALTERNATIVES

KALE WALDORF SALAD (V)

1 apple, cored and sliced

juice of ½ a lemon

1 stick of celery, sliced

1 scallion, finely sliced

2 handfuls of kale, washed, stems removed and finely sliced

⅓ cup walnuts, roughly chopped

FOR THE DRESSING

2 tablespoons dairy-free coconut yogurt or vegan mayonnaise

zest and juice of ½ a lemon

1 teaspoon whole-grain mustard

a pinch of sea salt and freshly ground black pepper, to taste

1 tablespoon extra-virgin olive oil

a few leaves of fresh tarragon, finely sliced (optional but does add a lovely layer of flavor)

PYRAMID:

This vegan Waldorf (the original uses mayonnaise) is still creamy and delicious, but definitely benefits from being made the night before—so the kale can soften and the dressing flavors can meld together (although add the walnuts just before serving or they can turn a little bitter). If you are making it on the day, you might prefer to use a more tender leaf, such as spinach, instead.

_____

Toss the apple slices in a bowl with the lemon juice so they don't brown, then remove, and mix with the celery, scallion, and kale.

Whisk the dressing ingredients together and toss through the salad so that it's evenly coated.

Add the chopped walnuts just before serving.

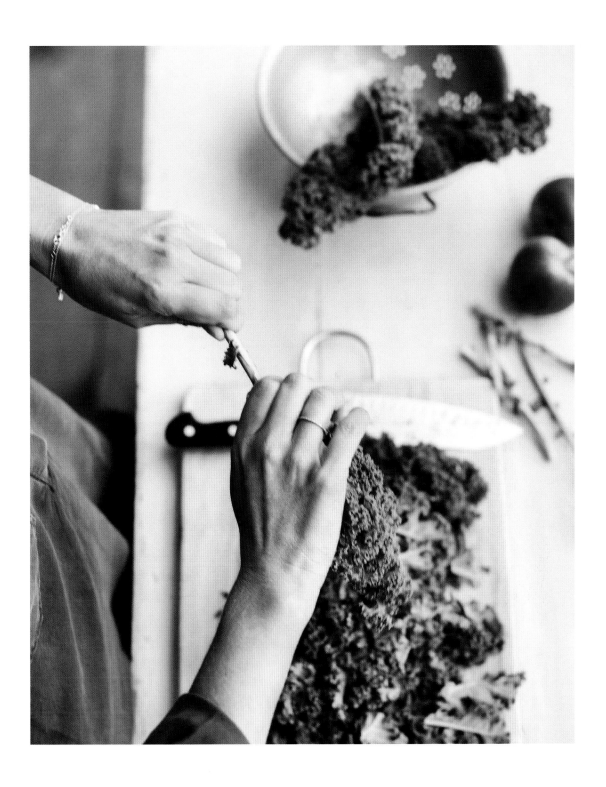

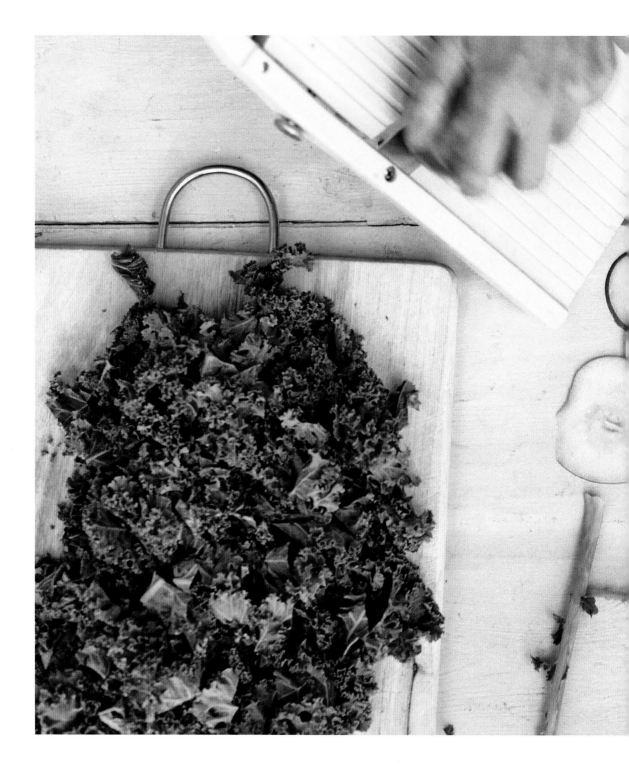

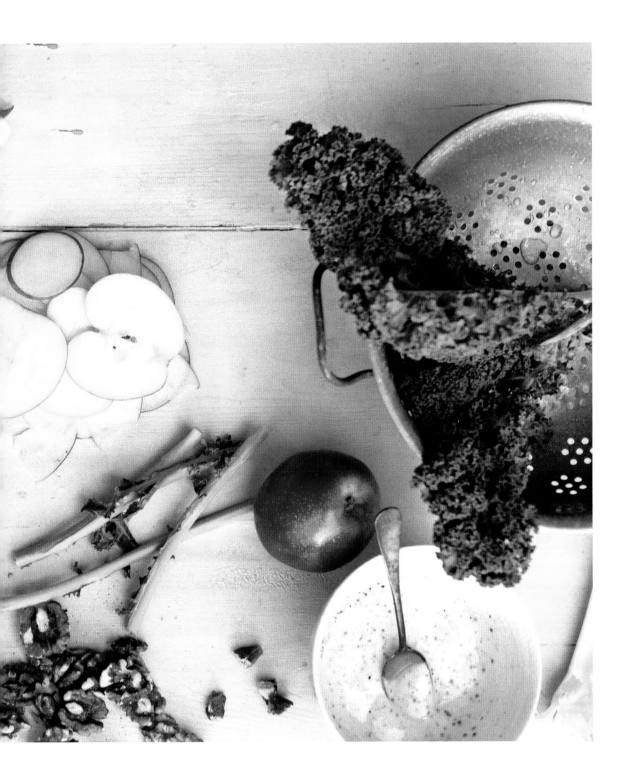

CHOPPED SALAD with SWEET POTATO FRIES (V)

11 oz sweet potatoes, washed

1 tablespoon light olive oil

½ teaspoon ground cumin

½ teaspoon ground coriander

FOR THE CHOPPED SALAD
(makes 2 portions)

1 x 14 oz can of black beans, drained and rinsed

1 red pepper, seeds removed and diced

heaping ½ cup sweet corn

1 stick of celery, finely diced

2 ripe medium tomatoes, finely diced

4-inch piece of cucumber, seeded and finely diced

2 tablespoons finely chopped fresh parsley or other fresh herbs (optional)

TO SERVE

2 tablespoons Tahini Dressing (see page 225)

a large wedge of lemon

¼ of an avocado, peeled and sliced

2 tablespoons Quick Pickled Cabbage (see page 224)

PYRAMID: 4

I think we all need a good chopped salad up our sleeves. It is simply a mixture of lots of delicious raw vegetables, prepared in a way that means that every mouthful gives you a combination not only of their unique flavors, but their textures too. Black beans are a great source of protein for vegans and vegetarians.

———————————

Preheat the oven to 400°F.

Chop half the sweet potatoes into wedges. Coat with the olive oil and the spices, and season well. Spread out on one half of a baking tray.

Peel the remaining sweet potatoes, chop into chunks, and coat with olive oil. Spread onto the other half of the baking tray. These will be used to make the frittata you'll have for breakfast tomorrow.

Put into the oven for 30–35 minutes, or until cooked through and starting to brown around the edges.

Meanwhile, mix together all the ingredients for the chopped salad. Season with salt and pepper. Set aside half for lunch tomorrow.

Once the chips are done, serve them alongside the rest of the salad with a generous portion of tahini dressing, the wedge of lemon to squeeze over the salad, some slices of ripe avocado, and a spoonful or two of tangy pickled cabbage.

Place the peeled sweet potato chunks into a bowl to cool down.

COMPLETE TODAY'S PREPARATION

after supper

1. Use the leftover peeled sweet potato chunks from supper tonight to make the Pea & Sweet Potato Fritter (see page 239) for breakfast tomorrow.

2. Use the leftover chicken and chopped salad from supper tonight to make your Chopped Chicken Salad for lunch tomorrow (see page 240).

for the vegan plan

1. *Use the leftover peeled sweet potato chunks from supper tonight to make the Pea & Sweet Potato Fritter (see page 246) for breakfast tomorrow.*

2. *Use the leftover chopped salad from supper tonight to make the Chopped Black Bean Salad for lunch tomorrow (see page 247).*

Mindful Moment

Pick one meal tomorrow where you know you will not be rushed. Put your fork down between each bite. This will encourage you to eat more slowly and more consciously, allowing time for your body's cues to reach your brain to let you know you are nearly full.

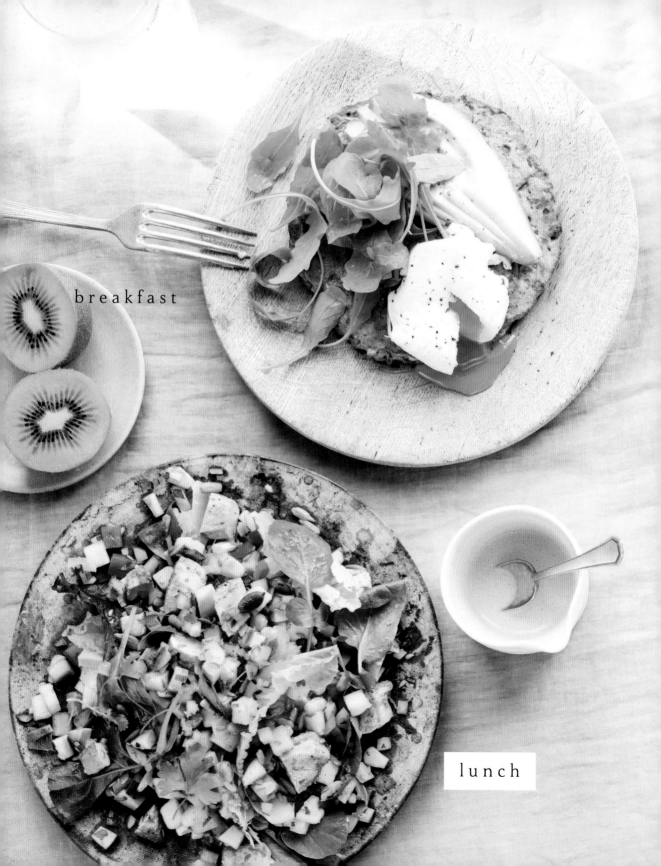

breakfast

lunch

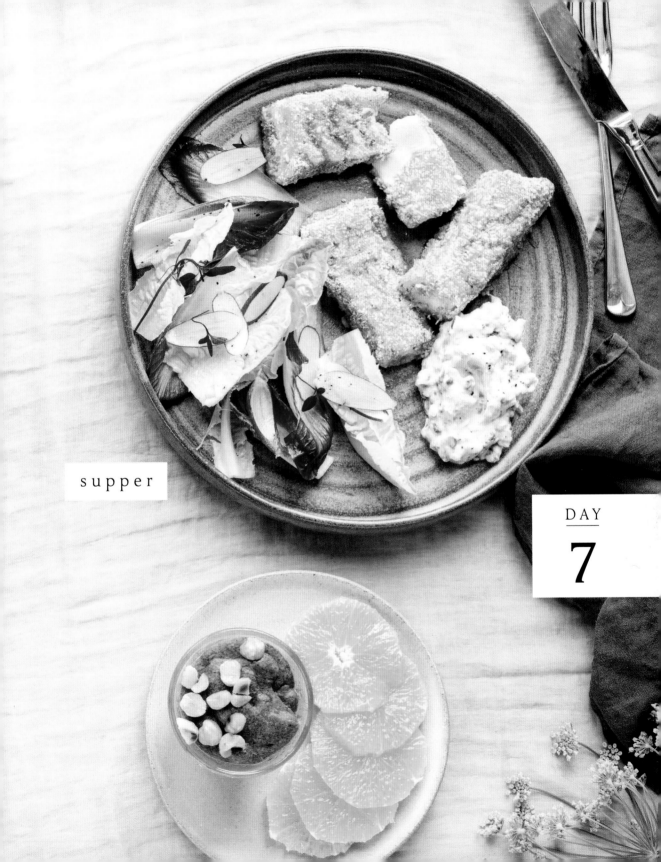

supper

DAY 7

BREAKFAST: PEA & SWEET POTATO FRITTER with a POACHED EGG + 1 PORTION of SEASONAL FRUIT

LUNCH: CHOPPED CHICKEN SALAD

SUPPER: FISH GOUJONS with TARTAR SAUCE + NUTTY CHOCOLATE POT

---

vegan alternatives:

BREAKFAST: PEA & SWEET POTATO FRITTER with AVOCADO + 1 PORTION of SEASONAL FRUIT

LUNCH: CHOPPED BLACK BEAN SALAD

SUPPER: FALAFEL BURGERS with a PORTOBELLO MUSHROOM "BUN" + NUTTY CHOCOLATE POT

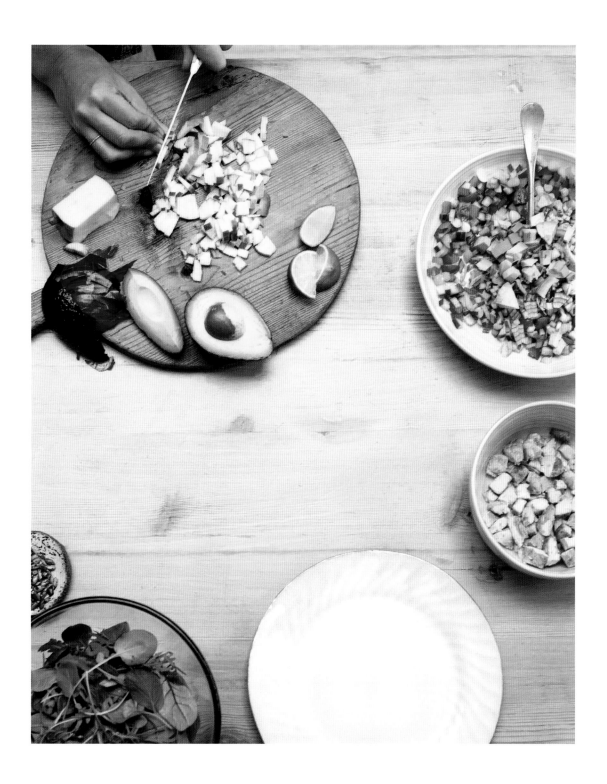

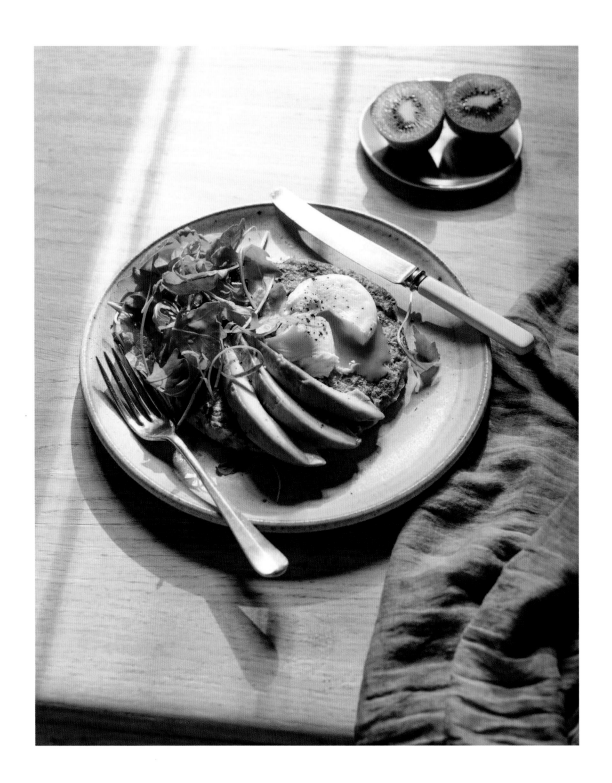

PEA & SWEET POTATO FRITTER

PYRAMID: **2** **1** **1** **2**

Fritters can be made with pretty much any vegetable and often contain some kind of flour, but I find they work best simply with leftover cooked potatoes or root vegetables.

a small handful of frozen peas

1¼ cups leftover cooked sweet potato chunks

1 scallion, finely sliced

1 tablespoon finely chopped fresh parsley (optional)

zest of ½ a lemon

sea salt and freshly ground black pepper

1 egg

coconut or light olive oil, for frying

TO SERVE

1 poached or soft-boiled egg

¼ of an avocado, peeled and sliced

a handful of arugula or salad leaves of your choice

In a heatproof bowl, cover the peas with boiling water for 4–5 minutes to defrost, then drain well.

Mash the leftover potatoes and peas with the back of a fork, then stir in the scallion, parsley, lemon zest, salt, and pepper. Whisk the egg, add it to the mix and stir through. You can prepare up to this step the night before and leave the mixture in the fridge overnight if you know you will be busy in the morning.

When you're ready to cook, place a frying pan over a medium heat and add a drizzle of oil. Spoon the mixture into the center of the pan and flatten to create a patty about 4–5 inches across and ½–1 inch deep. Fry for 3–4 minutes each side, or until heated through and starting to turn golden brown.

Meanwhile, poach or boil the other egg to your liking, and serve on top of the fritter, alongside the avocado and salad leaves.

CHOPPED CHICKEN SALAD

PYRAMID: 3

Chopped salads give a lovely mixture of textures and tastes all in one mouthful, not to mention being an excellent way to make use of lots of different vegetables. In this one I have thrown in some leftover chicken, and I've also added in an apple for a little sweetness. A delicious lunch, and the perfect fuel for a busy afternoon.

1 portion of leftover chicken (see page 222), roughly chopped

1 portion of leftover chopped salad (see page 222)

a handful of salad leaves of your choice

1 apple, cored and chopped

¼ of an avocado, peeled and chopped (optional)

½ a red onion, peeled and diced

2–3 tablespoons Spiced Seed Sprinkle (see page 140)

2 tablespoons Tahini Dressing (see page 225)

½ a lime, to squeeze on top

a few fresh cilantro leaves (optional)

Mix the chicken with the chopped salad and leaves and add the apple, avocado, red onion, and seed mix.

Keep the dressing separate until you serve the salad, then squeeze the lime juice on top and add a few extra cilantro leaves to garnish if you are using them.

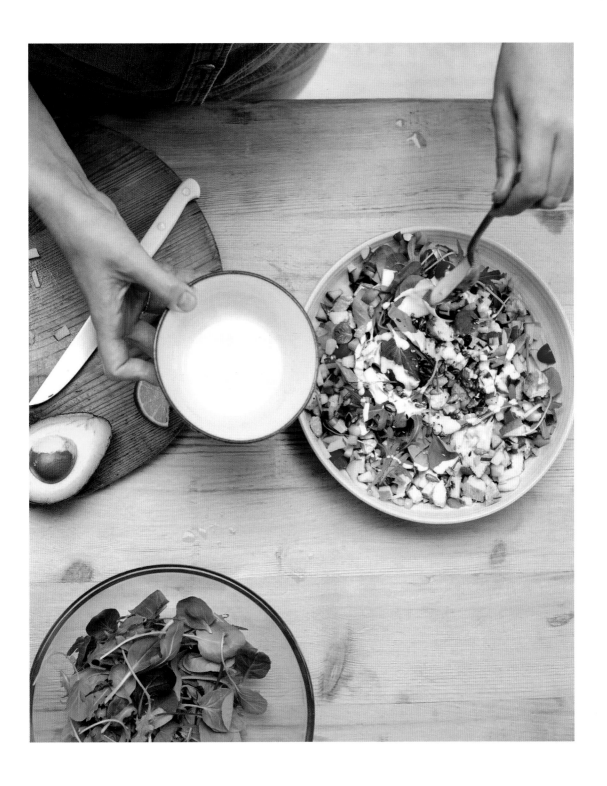

FISH GOUJONS with TARTAR SAUCE

light olive oil, melted coconut oil, or avocado oil

1 fillet of white fish

3 tablespoons gluten-free oats

zest of 1 lemon

¼ teaspoon turmeric

½ teaspoon sea salt flakes

a generous grind of fresh black pepper

⅛ teaspoon cayenne, paprika, or chili powder

1 egg, beaten

FOR THE TARTAR SAUCE:

1–2 tablespoons dairy-free coconut yogurt (or 1 tablespoon full-fat organic mayonnaise)

zest of ½ a small lemon, and a squeeze of juice

1 teaspoon capers

½ a shallot (or ¼ of a small red onion), peeled and roughly chopped

1 teaspoon chopped fresh parsley

sea salt and freshly ground black pepper

TO SERVE

2 big handfuls of fresh salad leaves of your choice

PYRAMID:

The lemon-flavored oat coating used in this dish makes for a really tasty gluten-free crunch. It could be used for anything you'd like to have a coating on, such as homemade chicken nuggets or even veggies. Fish is a fantastically healthy food all around. It's naturally low in saturated fat, a good source of protein, and an important source of dietary vitamin D, which is essential for strong bones. Cod, pollock, or haddock work well here.

Preheat the oven to 425°F. Line a baking tray with parchment paper, then drizzle some oil over the top.

Cut the fish into finger-sized pieces.

In a food processor (ideally a small spice grinder or NutriBullet with milling blade), grind the oats, lemon zest, turmeric, salt, pepper, and cayenne. Tip this onto a plate or into a shallow bowl. Beat the egg in another shallow bowl.

This part can get messy! Dip the fish pieces into the egg, then roll in the oat coating to cover all sides and transfer each piece to the lined and oiled baking tray. Continue this dipping and rolling until you've finished all the fish. Drizzle a little more oil over the top.

Place in the oven and bake for 10 minutes, then use a spatula to turn the pieces over and bake for a further 3–5 minutes.

While the fish is cooking, make the tartar sauce by pulsing all the ingredients together in a small blender a couple of times, leaving it a little bit chunky.

Check that the fish is cooked (it should be white all the way through). Serve with the tartar sauce and fresh green salad leaves on the side.

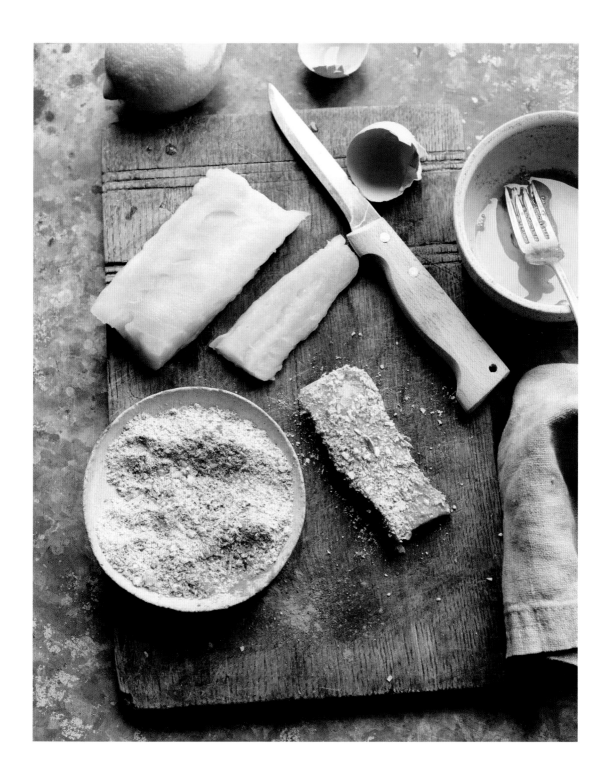

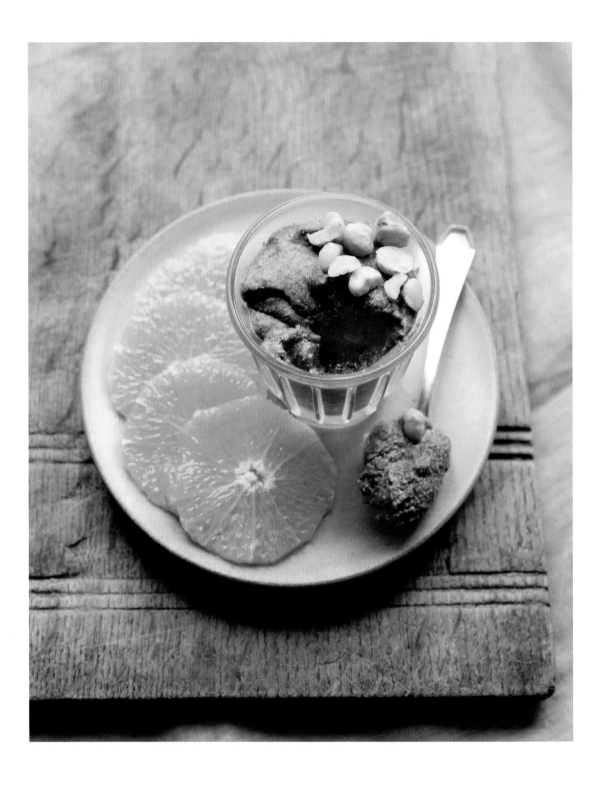

NUTTY CHOCOLATE POT (V)

PYRAMID:

This tastes like an indulgent chocolate mousse, yet is much easier to make. I hope this will become one of your go-to desserts for those moments when you fancy something rich and chocolatey, or to serve to any lucky dinner guests that you may be entertaining. Cocoa is one of our best dietary sources of polyphenols, and has been linked to improved brain function, healthy aging, and heart benefits. However, it is the cocoa (or cacao) content that is important, so when cooking or eating chocolate, look for something with 85 percent cocoa content minimum.

scant ¼ cup hazelnuts or almonds

1 tablespoon chia seeds

½ cup canned full-fat coconut milk (about ½ a can)

1 tablespoon sweetener of choice (such as honey or maple syrup)

½ teaspoon organic vanilla extract

2 heaped teaspoons raw cacao powder (or organic cocoa powder)

TO SERVE

Fresh fruit of your choice

Toast the hazelnuts or almonds in a dry frying pan over medium heat for 1–2 minutes each side, stirring regularly. Watch them carefully—they have a tendency to burn if left alone! Once done, turn them on to a board and roughly chop.

Combine the rest of the ingredients in a blender and whizz on high speed until smooth. Stir half the chopped nuts through the mix, and spoon into a small glass. Top with the remaining nuts and leave in the fridge to set for at least 30 minutes, ideally longer if you have the time. Serve with a portion of fruit alongside. Fresh orange segments or a bowl of fresh raspberries are particularly delicious!

VARIATIONS   Here are a few suggestions for alternatives, but let your imagination run wild!

- Add 3 or 4 fresh mint leaves before blending for a mint-chocolate pot
- Add the zest of ½ a small orange and a couple of tablespoons of orange juice to the mix
- Stir through 1 tablespoon of raw cacao nibs for a double-chocolate hit
- Add ½ teaspoon of ground cinnamon and ¼ teaspoon of grated nutmeg before blending for a wintry spiced-chocolate variation

VEGAN ALTERNATIVES

PEA & SWEET POTATO FRITTER (V)

PYRAMID:

This delicious breakfast is really simple to make and I hope it will become a firm favorite in your vegan recipe repertoire. Using chia seeds (instead of an egg) as the binding agent helps to hold the fritter together during frying, allowing it to become golden and crisp on the outside while still staying soft on the inside. Adding in some avocado for healthy fats and a sprinkling of toasted seeds for extra protein makes this a lovely, balanced vegan brekkie.

½ tablespoon chia seeds

a small handful of frozen peas

1¼ cups leftover cooked sweet potato chunks

1 scallion, finely sliced

1 tablespoon finely chopped fresh parsley (optional)

zest of ½ a lemon

sea salt and freshly ground black pepper

coconut or light olive oil, for frying

TO SERVE

a handful of arugula or salad leaves of your choice

½ an avocado, peeled and sliced

2–3 tablespoons Spiced Seed Sprinkle (see page 140)

Mix the chia seeds with 2 tablespoons of water and leave to rest for 10 minutes or so, until thick and goopy.

In a heatproof bowl, cover the peas with boiling water for 4–5 minutes to defrost, then drain well.

Mash the leftover potato and peas together with the back of a fork, then stir in the scallion, parsley, lemon zest, salt, and pepper.

Add the chia seed mixture and stir through. You can prepare up to this step the night before, and leave the mixture in the fridge overnight if you know you will be busy in the morning.

When you're ready to cook, place a frying pan over medium heat and add a drizzle of oil. Spoon the mixture into the center of the pan and flatten to create a patty about 4–5 inches across and 1 inch deep. Fry for 5 minutes each side, or until heated through and starting to turn golden brown.

Serve the fritter on a bed of salad leaves, with some thinly sliced avocado and a generous sprinkling of toasted seeds.

CHOPPED BLACK BEAN SALAD (V)

PYRAMID:

This should be a very quick lunch to put together, as you will have already made the chopped salad for supper on Day 6. It's jazzed up a little here with some sweet apple, crunchy red onion, and smooth avocado. This is exactly the sort of thing that I eat really regularly—simple, tasty, and nutritious.

1 apple, cored and chopped

½ a small red onion, peeled and diced (optional)

¼ of an avocado, peeled and chopped

1 portion of leftover chopped salad (see page 232)

½ a lime, to squeeze on top

a handful of salad leaves of your choice

2 tablespoons Spiced Seed Sprinkle (see page 140)

a few fresh cilantro leaves (optional)

2 tablespoons Tahini Dressing (see page 225)

Mix the apple, red onion, and avocado into your leftover chopped salad. Add a squeeze of lime juice and stir it through to help prevent anything from browning. (You might want to keep the avocado separate from the salad if you are preparing it ahead of time, and add it at the last minute. It can look a little discolored if prepared and left overnight.)

To serve, spoon the chopped salad over some salad leaves, sprinkle on some seeds, and top with a few cilantro leaves. Drizzle with the tahini dressing just before eating.

FALAFEL BURGERS (V)

FOR THE FALAFEL
(makes 2 portions)

½ tablespoon chia seeds

1 x 14 oz can of chickpeas, drained and rinsed

1 scallion, chopped

1 clove of garlic, peeled and roughly chopped

2 teaspoons ground cumin

½ teaspoon sea salt

2 tablespoons roughly chopped fresh parsley

juice of ½ a lemon

light olive oil, for brushing

TO SERVE

2 portobello mushrooms, stems removed and brushed clean

2 tablespoons Tahini Dressing (see page 225)

1–2 tomatoes, sliced

a large handful of crispy lettuce leaves

2 tablespoons Quick Pickled Cabbage (see page 224)

PYRAMID:

Chickpeas, like all legumes, are a source of plant-based protein as well as fiber and complex carbohydrates. They are therefore filling and nutritious, and deliciously tasty to eat. I love using them in loaded-up portobello mushroom "buns"—a great way to get your burger fix while still fully nourishing your health.

Mix the chia seeds with 2 tablespoons of water, and leave to rest for 10 minutes or so, until thick and goopy.

Place this, along with all the other falafel ingredients, into a food processor, and blend until smooth—about 30 seconds or so.

With lightly oiled hands, make 2 firm patties, roughly 2–3 inches wide. Place them in the fridge for at least 30 minutes to chill, as this helps them to hold together while cooking.

After they have chilled, turn your broiler to medium-hot. Place the patties and mushroom halves (gills facing upward) onto a large oiled baking tray, brush both with a little olive oil, and broil for 8–10 minutes or until lightly golden brown. Remove the tray from under the broiler, flip over the patties and mushrooms, brushing the other side with a little more oil, and broil for a further 6–8 minutes.

Place one falafel in between the two grilled mushroom halves. Drizzle over some tahini dressing, then load up with juicy tomato slices, crispy lettuce, and pickled cabbage.

Leave the leftover patty in the fridge for lunch tomorrow.

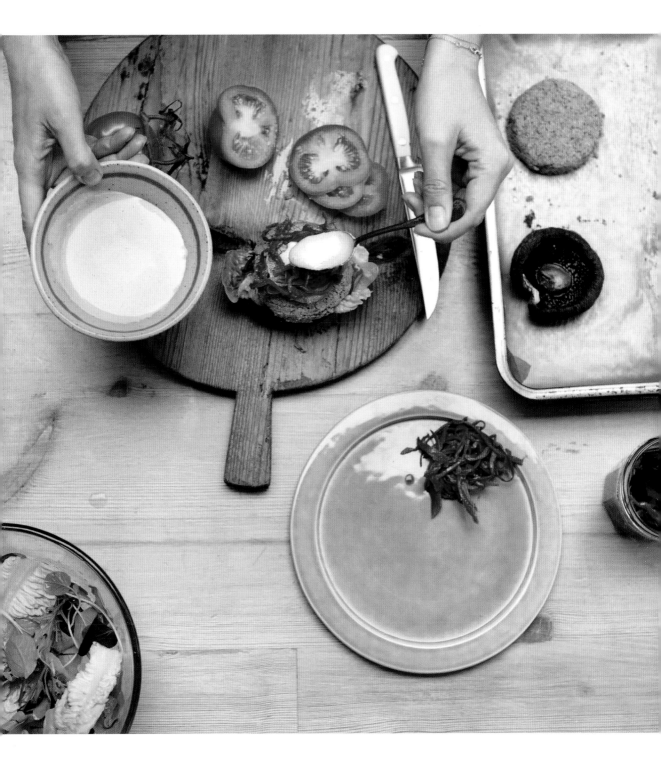

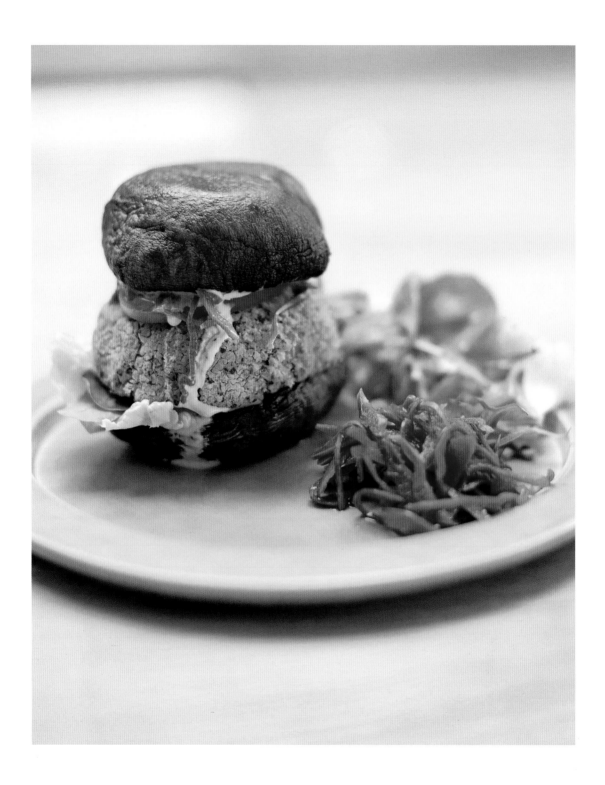

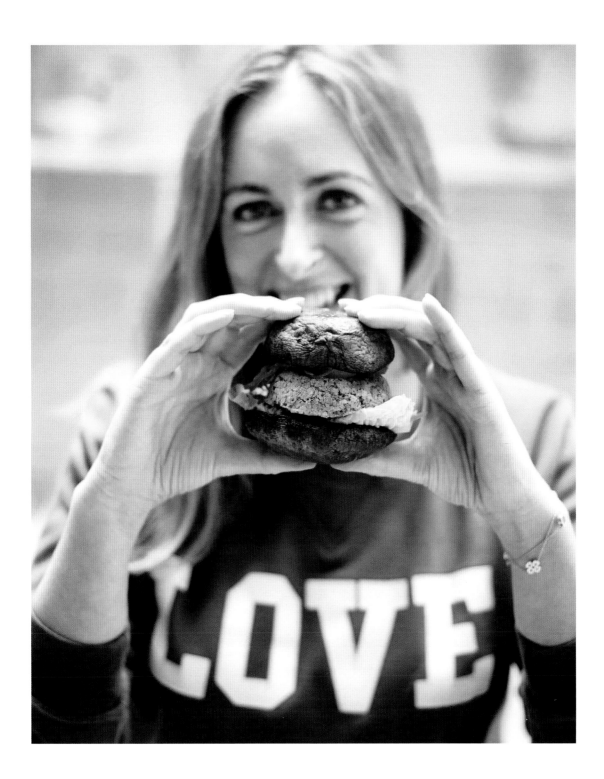

COMPLETE TODAY'S PREPARATION

after supper

1. Prepare the ingredients for the Herby Green Omelet (see page 259) for breakfast tomorrow.

2. Make the Smoked Salmon Pâté (see page 260) and prepare some raw vegetable crudités for lunch tomorrow.

for the vegan plan

1. *Roast the tomatoes and prepare the kale for the Sweet Potato Toasts with Scrambled Tofu for breakfast tomorrow (see page 267).*

2. *Prepare your Falafel Salad (see page 270) for lunch tomorrow and leave it in the fridge overnight.*

Mindful Moment

Take a moment after each of your meals tomorrow to think about to how it made you *feel*. Are you comfortably full, stuffed, or do you feel you need to eat more? Do you feel energized or lethargic? Did you enjoy the experience of preparing and eating that meal? Do you have any other symptoms (like bloating or abdominal pain)? Is there anything your body is trying to tell you right now? If so, listen carefully to it.

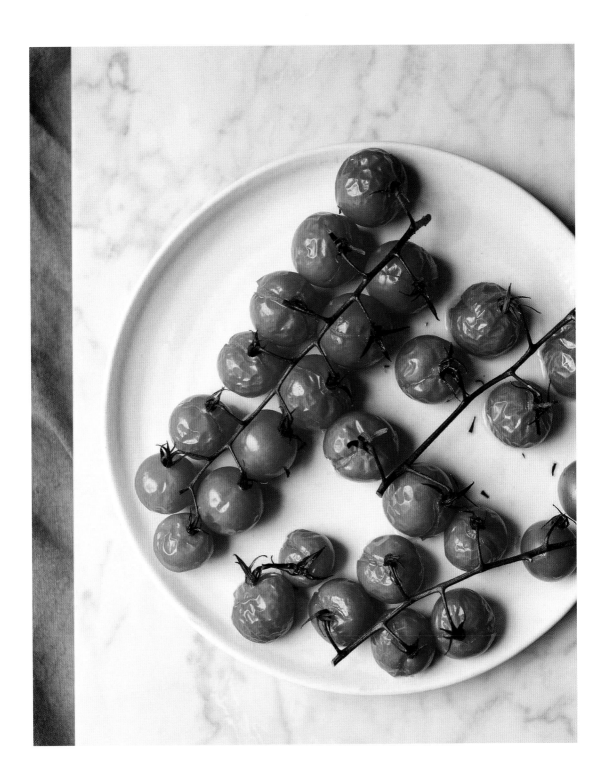

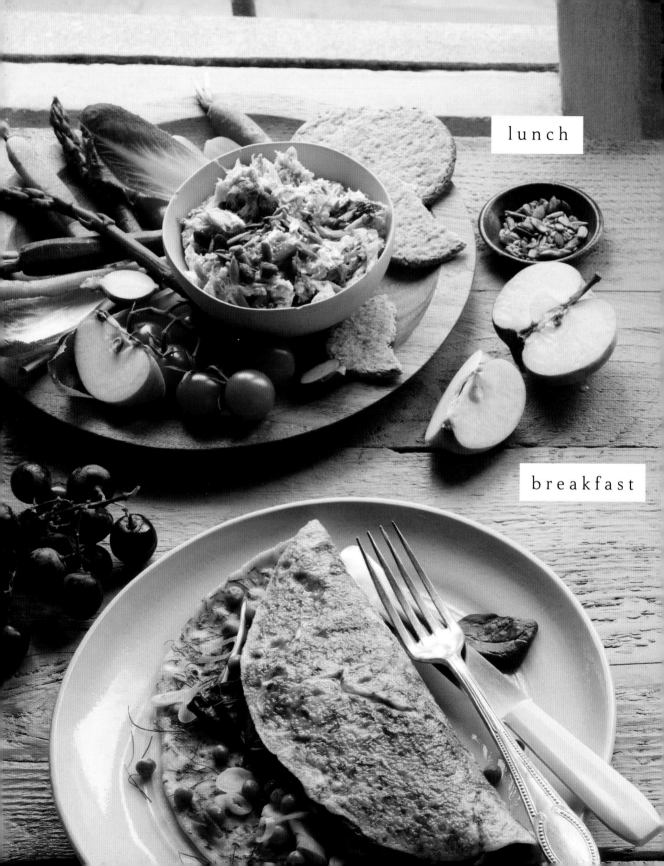

lunch

breakfast

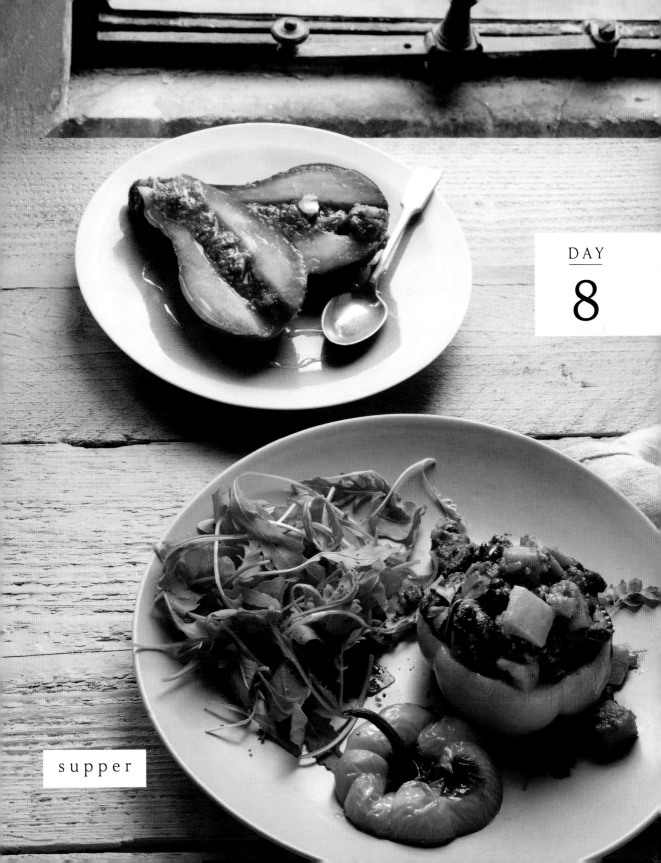

DAY

8

supper

DAY 8

BREAKFAST: HERBY GREEN OMELET
+ 1 PORTION of SEASONAL FRUIT

LUNCH: SMOKED SALMON PÂTÉ with
VEGETABLE CRUDITÉS and OATCAKES
+ 1 PORTION of SEASONAL FRUIT

SUPPER: STUFFED PEPPERS with CHILI (v)
+ BAKED ORANGE & ALMOND PEAR

vegan alternatives:

BREAKFAST: SWEET POTATO TOASTS with
SCRAMBLED TOFU, ROASTED TOMATOES, and KALE
+ 1 PORTION of SEASONAL FRUIT

LUNCH: FALAFEL SALAD
+ 1 PORTION of SEASONAL FRUIT

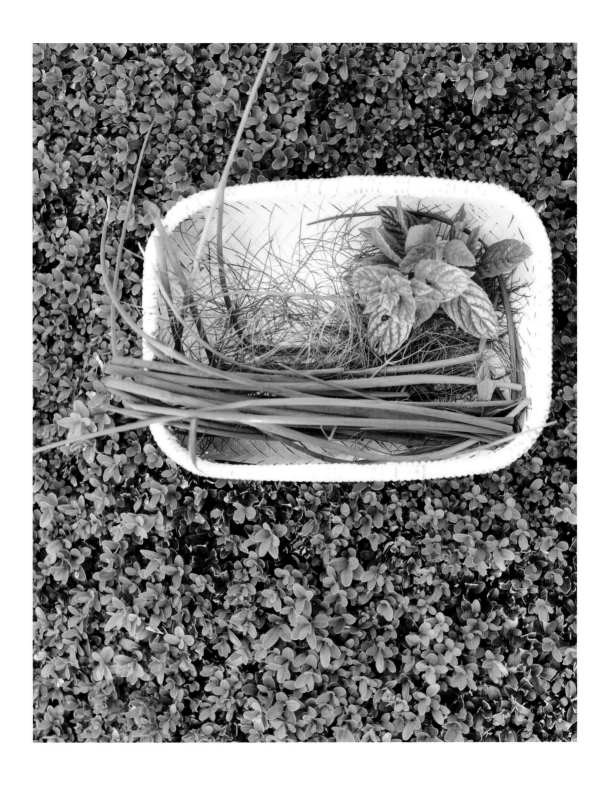

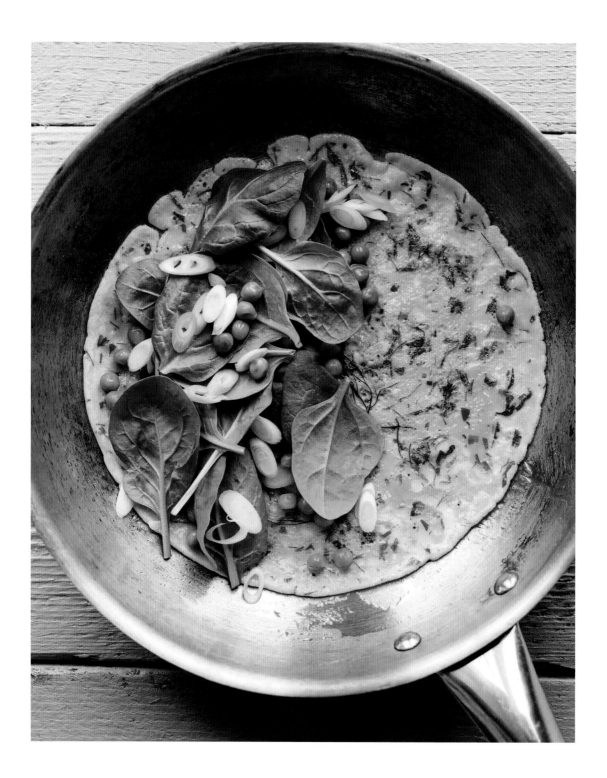

HERBY GREEN OMELET

PYRAMID: 1

This is a super-fast breakfast, filled with fresh herby greens. It will cook in about 3 minutes, so make sure you have all your ingredients chopped and ready before you heat the pan up. Try experimenting with different herbs too: cilantro, chives, basil, arugula, and even mint can also work well. Just choose whatever you have to hand, growing, or is in season.

2 large eggs, preferably free-range or organic

sea salt and freshly ground black pepper

2 tablespoons finely chopped fresh parsley and/or dill

1 tablespoon coconut oil or light olive oil

2 scallions, finely sliced

2 handfuls of spinach

a handful of peas (if frozen, pour boiling water over them in a small bowl to thaw for 5 minutes, then drain)

In a small bowl, whisk the eggs with a pinch of salt, a grind of fresh black pepper, and the chopped fresh herbs, either dill or parsley (or both).

Heat the coconut oil or olive oil in a wide frying pan over medium heat, making sure the base of the pan is coated so your eggs don't stick. Add the eggs and swirl again so you have a thin coating—it should bubble just slightly at the edges. Keep tilting the pan to distribute the egg evenly.

Sprinkle with the scallions, spinach, and peas, and cook for about 2 minutes, until the egg is almost dry, then fold over just under half of the egg to cover the greens, leaving a smile of green showing. Cook for 1 minute more, then slide the omelet out of the pan and onto your plate.

SMOKED SALMON PÂTÉ

3½ oz smoked salmon, skin and bones removed

zest and juice of ½ a lime

3 tablespoons finely chopped fresh cilantro

1 fresh red chili pepper, seeded and finely chopped

1-inch piece of fresh ginger, peeled and finely grated

2 tablespoons dairy-free coconut yogurt (or 1 tablespoon full-fat organic mayonnaise)

1 tablespoon coconut aminos

2 scallions, finely sliced

sea salt and black pepper, to taste

TO SERVE

2 or 3 gluten-free oatcakes

1 apple, sliced

3 portions of raw vegetable crudités (a handful of asparagus tips, some endive leaves, and ½ a sliced pepper, for example)

2 tablespoons Spiced Seed Sprinkle (see page 140)

PYRAMID:

This spicy, zingy take on classic smoked salmon pâté is a sure-fire hit. I love it in a bowl for lunch with lots of bits and pieces for dipping, but you could also pile it into lettuce cups, or even spread it on some gluten-free toast for an alternative breakfast.

Mix all the pâté ingredients together with a fork, tasting and seasoning accordingly.

Spoon the pâté into a bowl and serve with the oatcakes, sliced apple, vegetable crudités, and a generous sprinkling of toasted seeds.

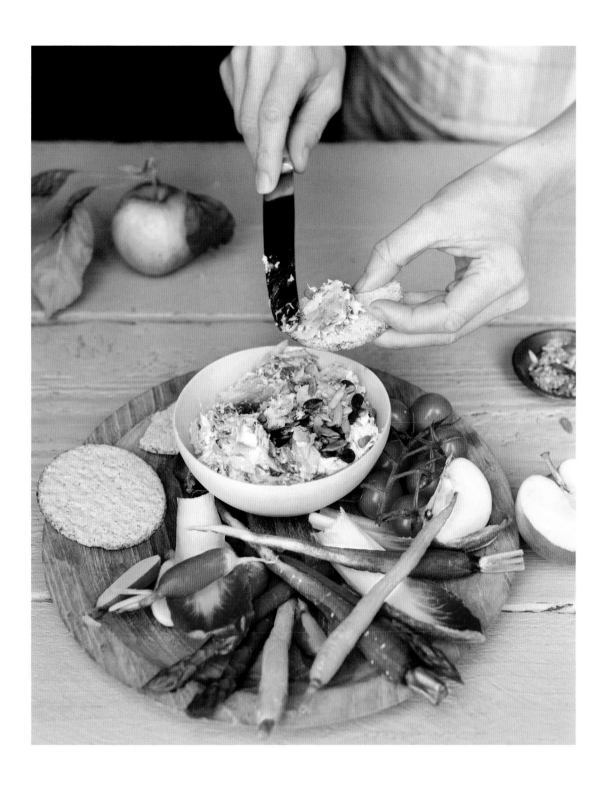

STUFFED PEPPERS with CHILI (V)

1 large red or yellow pepper

1 teaspoon light olive oil

FOR THE CHILI

1 teaspoon coconut oil or light olive oil

½ a small red onion, peeled and sliced

1 clove of garlic, peeled and sliced

1 small stick of celery, diced

½ a red chili pepper, diced

3.5 oz sweet potatoes, peeled and diced into ½–1 inch pieces

1 teaspoon ground cumin

1 teaspoon ground coriander

½ teaspoon paprika

a small bunch of fresh cilantro, stems finely chopped, leaves reserved

½ a 14 oz can of black beans or kidney beans, drained and rinsed

1 tablespoon tomato puree

PYRAMID: **4**

This hearty and warming vegan chili filling is a great recipe to have up your sleeve for those nights when you need a warming, healthy meal. It works well as a standalone dish too—just load up a bowl and add a handful of seasonal greens, or pour it over some brown rice for a filling supper after a long, blustery day out.

This bean and sweet potato chili is a very easy recipe to make a big batch of and freeze in portions, so you could always double up the quantities and put some away for another day (which will also prevent you from being left with half a can of beans looking sad in the fridge!).

Preheat the oven to 400°F.

Heat the oil in a saucepan and sauté the onion, garlic, celery, chili pepper, and sweet potatoes for 5 minutes, then stir in the ground cumin and ground coriander, paprika, and cilantro stalks until everything is well coated.

Add ½ cup of water and cover with a tight-fitting lid. Turn the heat down to its lowest setting and cook for 25–30 minutes, stirring occasionally to stop it from sticking.

Meanwhile, cut the pepper in half straight through the stalk and carefully take out the seeds and pithy white parts from inside. Pour ½ teaspoon of olive oil inside each half pepper and use your hands to rub this all over both sides. Place on a baking tray, skin side down, and put into the oven for 12–15 minutes, to soften. Remove from the oven when the peppers are soft and slightly caramelized around the edges, and set aside.

1 teaspoon tamari or coconut
aminos

sea salt and freshly ground
black pepper

TO SERVE

a handful of salad leaves of
your choice

After the filling has simmered for 25–30 minutes, add the beans, tomato puree and tamari. You may need to add another splash of water if it looks dry, although you are aiming for quite a thick mixture. Bring back to a simmer for another 5–6 minutes, to warm the beans through. Stir in half the cilantro leaves, then taste and adjust the seasoning as necessary.

Spoon the mixture into your prepared pepper halves, sprinkle with the remaining cilantro leaves, and serve over a bed of salad leaves of your choice.

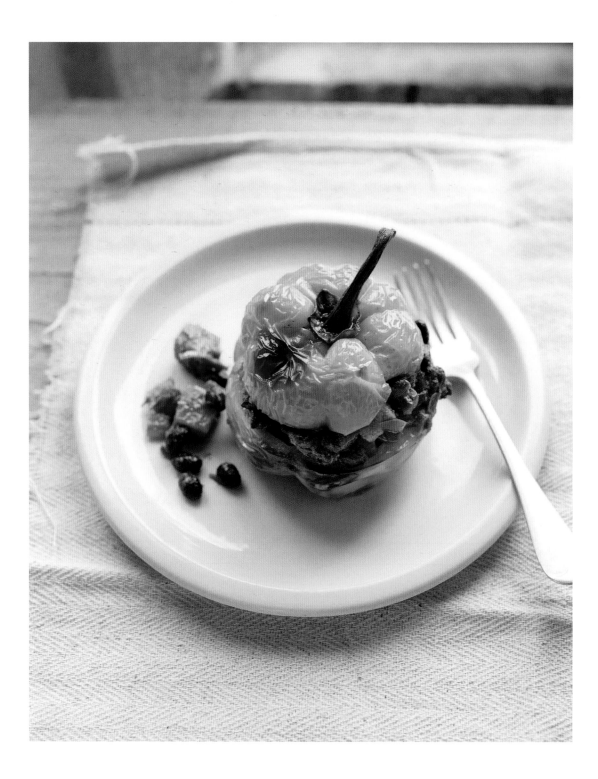

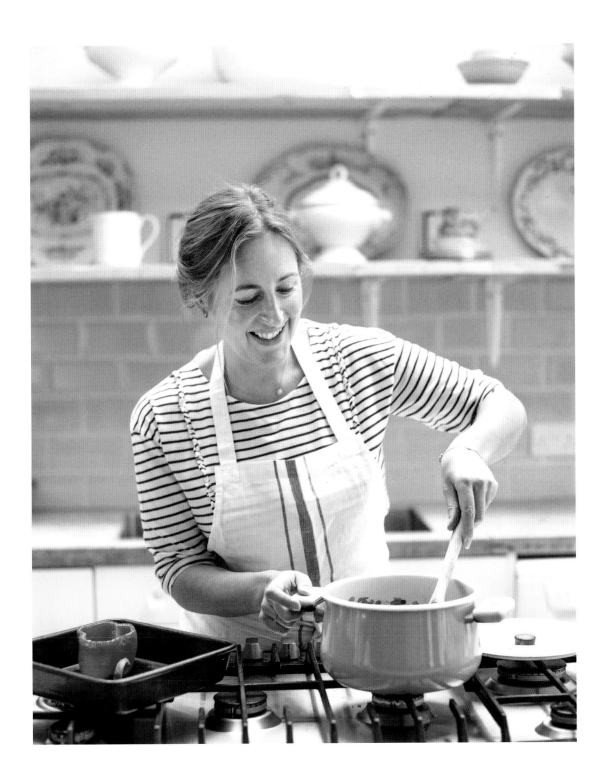

BAKED ORANGE & ALMOND PEAR (V)

MAKES: 2 portions

PYRAMID:

Stuffed with a mixture of zesty orange, flaxseeds (grinding them helps digestion and absorption), and crunchy almonds, these pears are a lovely dessert if you want one. The recipe works well for a crowd too—just multiply the quantities by the number of portions you need.

If you want, you could substitute apples for the pears, or swap the vanilla extract for 1 teaspoon of ground cinnamon for a warming, autumnal treat. Ground flaxseed can be found in most good supermarkets now.

2 small ripe pears, cored

12 almonds or hazelnuts, chopped

zest and juice of 1 small orange

2 tablespoons ground flaxseed

½ teaspoon organic vanilla extract

TO SERVE

1 teaspoon sweetener of choice (honey, maple syrup, or coconut nectar), drizzled on top just before serving

Preheat the oven to 400°F. You will need ramekins that fit the pears snugly.

Place the cored pears in the ramekins. In a bowl, mix the rest of the ingredients and spoon inside each pear—don't worry if some oozes out of the top. Sprinkle with 1–2 tablespoons of water and put into the oven for 18–20 minutes, or until a sharp knife slips into the pears without resistance.

Enjoy one while still warm tonight, drizzled with your sweetener of choice, and leave the other to cool for breakfast tomorrow morning.

VEGAN ALTERNATIVES

SWEET POTATO TOASTS
with SCRAMBLED TOFU (V)

PYRAMID:

Yes, sweet potato toast really does work! Naturally gluten-free and delicious toast with minimal effort. You can try it with all sorts of different toppings—mashed avocado, a pinch of chili flakes, and a sprinkling of toasted seeds is another favorite of mine.

6–8 cherry tomatoes,
on the vine

freshly ground black pepper

1 sweet potato, washed

2 tablespoons olive oil

1 clove of garlic, peeled and
finely chopped

5½ oz firm tofu, drained

¼ teaspoon ground turmeric

a generous pinch of sea salt
and freshly ground
black pepper

a handful of kale, stems
removed and finely sliced
(you could substitute spinach
or chard here too)

1 tablespoon pesto
(see page 211)

Preheat the oven to 400°F. Place the tomato vine onto a small baking tray, season with black pepper, and roast in the oven for 10 minutes. If you are strapped for time, feel free to just quarter the cherry tomatoes and have them raw instead.

Slice the sweet potato lengthwise into ½-inch slices. Place two slices straight into the toaster and toast 2–3 times, turning each time or until the flesh is tender when poked with a fork and the outside is lightly golden and slightly crisp.

Meanwhile, make the scrambled tofu. Heat 1 tablespoon of olive oil in a small pan, add the garlic, and cook over gentle heat for 30 seconds. Add the tofu to the pan, breaking it up into small pieces with a wooden spoon.

Add the turmeric, salt, and pepper and cook over medium heat for 2 minutes. Add 1 tablespoon of hot water and stir until it has all been incorporated.

Steam the kale and allow to wilt for 1–2 minutes in a separate pan. Drizzle with 1 tablespoon of olive oil.

To serve, place 2 slices of sweet potato toast on a serving plate, top with the scrambled tofu and roasted cherry tomatoes, and add a dollop of pesto. Serve with the kale alongside.

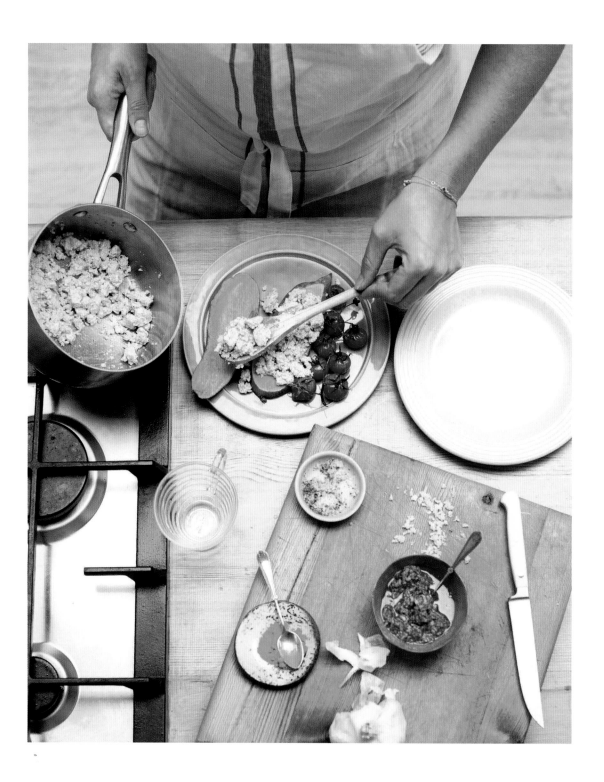

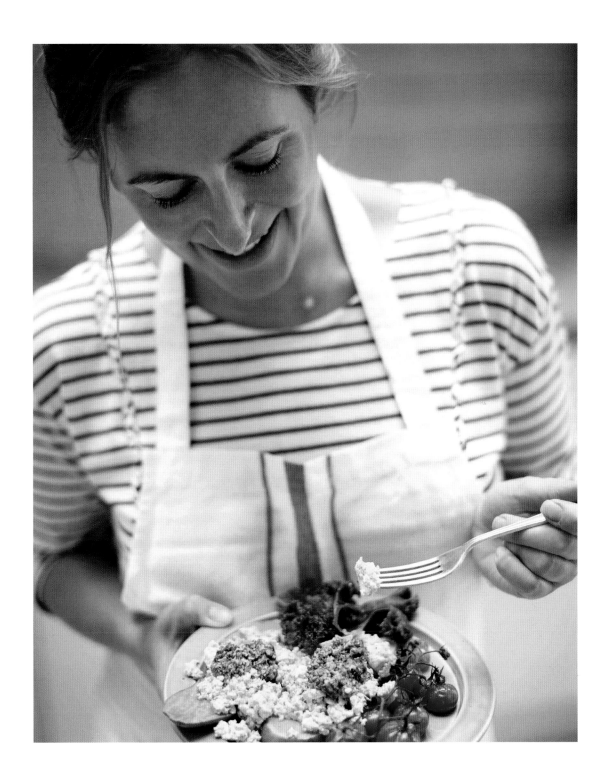

FALAFEL SALAD (V)

a handful of baby leaf salad (with chopped herbs if you have some)

1 large carrot, peeled and grated

4-inch piece of cucumber, diced

¼ of an avocado, peeled and diced

7–8 cherry tomatoes

1 tablespoon Spiced Seed Sprinkle (see page 140)

1 leftover falafel patty (see page 248)

a drizzle of extra-virgin olive oil

a dash of apple cider vinegar

2 tablespoons Tahini Dressing (see page 225)

PYRAMID:

Arrange the vegetables in a bowl or lunchbox. Sprinkle over the seeds and arrange the falafel patty on top.

The falafel is delicious cold, but you could always warm it through slightly before serving.

Drizzle the salad with olive oil and vinegar just before serving and add a dollop of tahini dressing on top of the patty.

COMPLETE TODAY'S PREPARATION

after supper

1. Leave the second pear to cool down fully then put it in the fridge overnight, ready for breakfast tomorrow morning.

2. Prepare the Italian Tuna Salad for lunch tomorrow (see page 279).

for the vegan plan

1. *Leave the second pear to cool down fully then put it in the fridge overnight, ready for breakfast tomorrow morning.*

2. *Prepare the Green Bean, Pea & Pistachio Salad for lunch tomorrow (see page 282).*

Mindful Moment

Focus on the following phrase tomorrow: *savor every single bite*. If necessary, say it to yourself out loud before starting each meal.

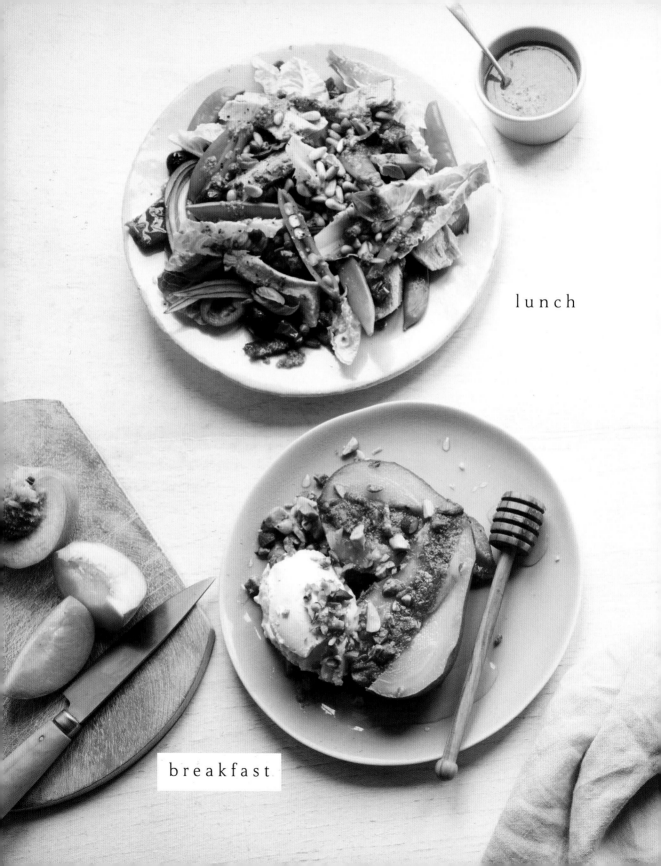

lunch

breakfast

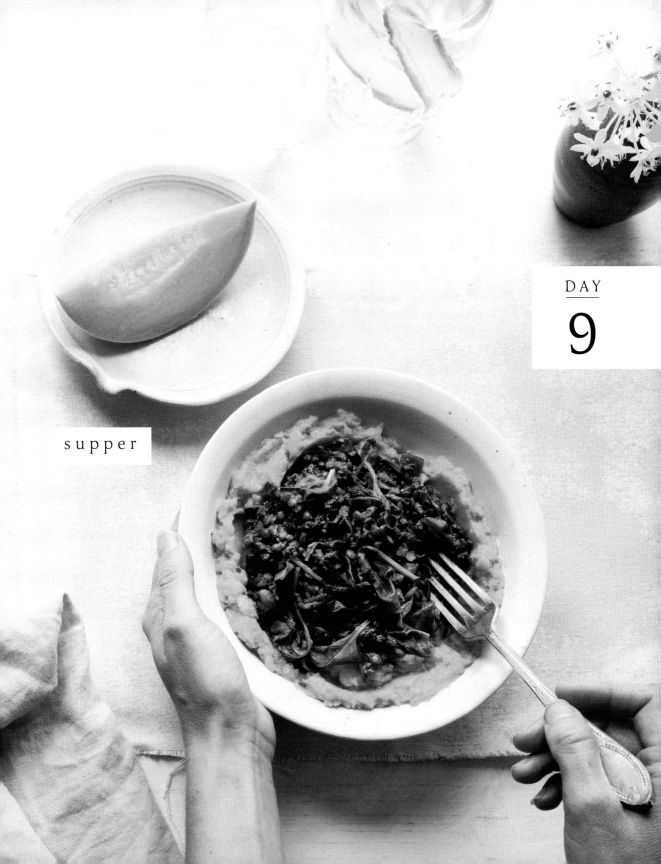

supper

DAY 9

BREAKFAST: BAKED PEAR BREAKFAST BOWL (v)

LUNCH: ITALIAN TUNA SALAD
+ 1 PORTION of SEASONAL FRUIT

SUPPER: COTTAGE PIE
+ 1 PORTION of SEASONAL FRUIT

---

vegan alternatives:

LUNCH: GREEN BEAN, PEA & PISTACHIO SALAD
+ 1 PORTION of SEASONAL FRUIT

SUPPER: LENTIL "COTTAGE" PIE
+ 1 PORTION of SEASONAL FRUIT

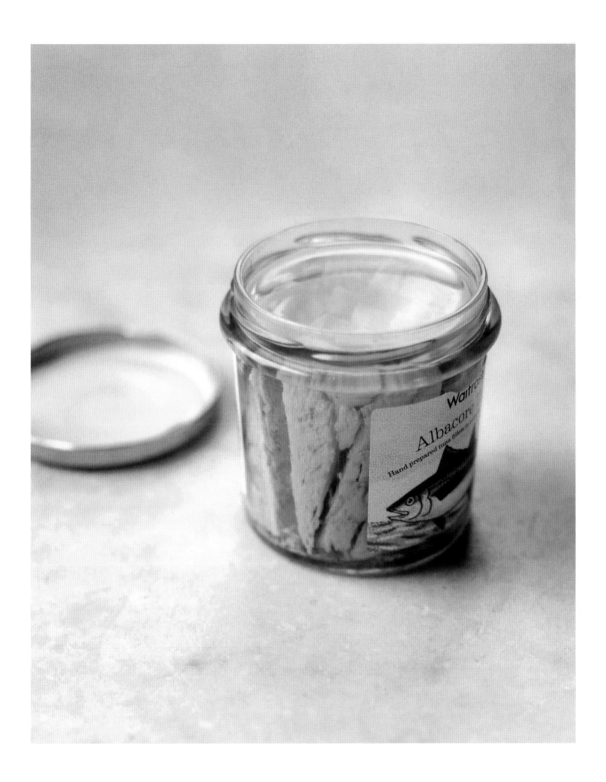

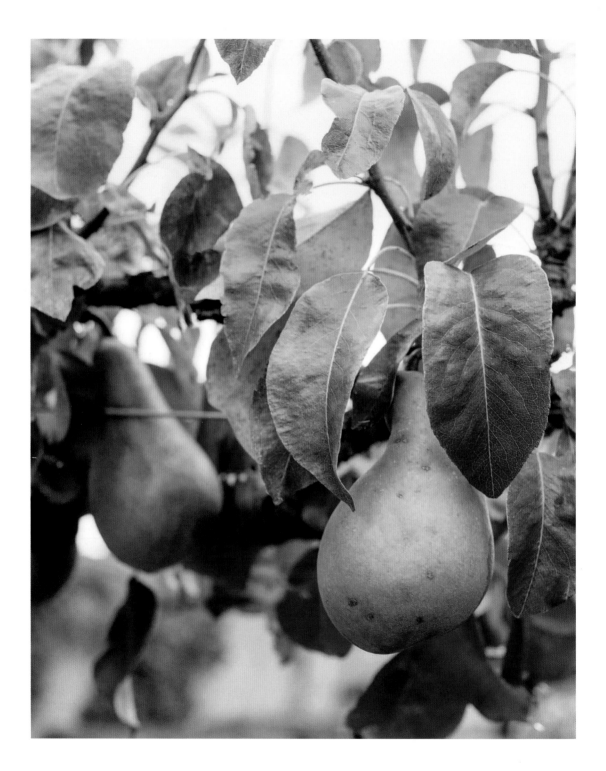

BAKED PEAR BREAKFAST BOWL (V)

1 leftover Baked Orange
& Almond Pear
(see page 266)

2–3 tablespoons dairy-free
coconut yogurt

3 tablespoons Nut Granola
(see page 141)

PYRAMID: 1

Serve your leftover baked pear with a dollop of coconut yogurt and some granola.

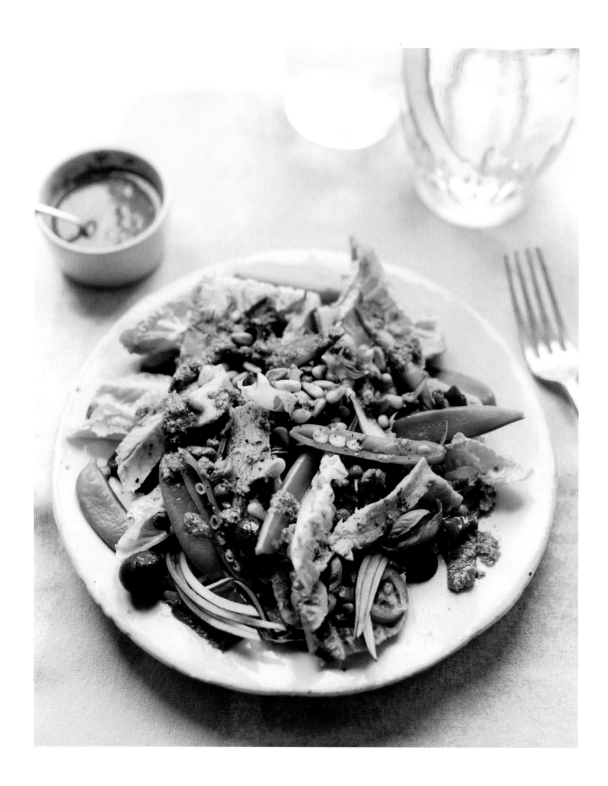

ITALIAN TUNA SALAD

1 cup sugar snap peas
(or green beans)

1 tablespoon pine nuts (you
could also use sunflower seeds)

3½ oz responsibly sourced
canned or jarred tuna

8–10 black olives

½ a red pepper, seeded and
sliced

¼ of a red onion, peeled
and very finely sliced

3 sun-dried tomatoes,
drained and chopped

a big handful of salad leaves
(I love Bibb or arugula here)

a few extra basil leaves,
for flavor (optional)

1 teaspoon capers (optional)

FOR THE PESTO *(see page 211)*

PYRAMID: **4**

This super simple salad is the type of thing that I eat most days. It can be thrown together in minutes from ingredients I almost always have lying around, and yet still packs both a nutritional and a flavor punch. Delicious.

Blanch the sugar snap peas by boiling or steaming them for 1–2 minutes. Drain immediately, then place under running cold water for a few seconds to stop the cooking.

If you like, you could also toast the pine nuts for a minute or so in a dry frying pan over medium heat to give them a little extra color. You could skip this step if you are pressed for time.

Put all the pesto ingredients into a small blender and blend for a minute or so, until well combined. If it looks a little dry, add an extra squeeze of lemon juice. This step can be done ahead of time—just put the pesto into a little jar, screw the lid on, and leave in the fridge overnight.

When you are ready to make the salad, pile all the salad ingredients on to a plate, sprinkle with the pine nuts and capers, and drizzle over some pesto.

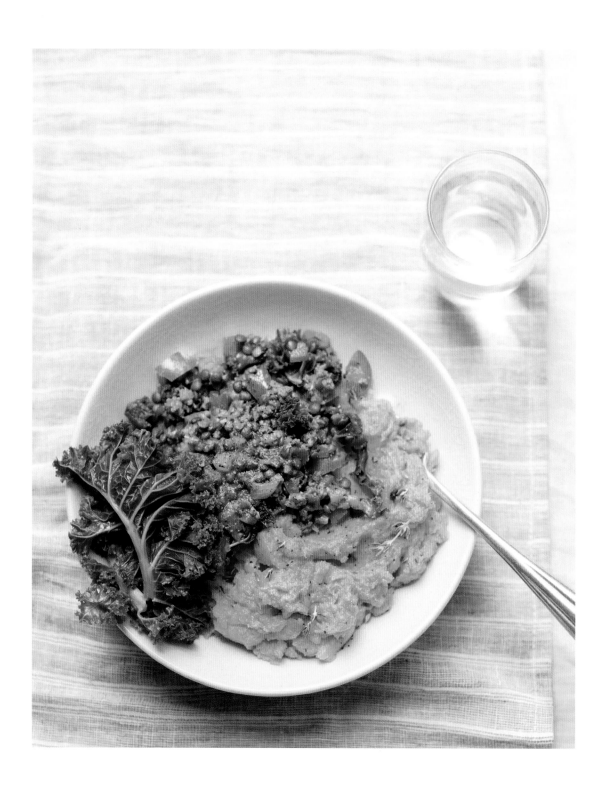

COTTAGE PIE

MAKES: 2 portions

1 tablespoon light olive oil

1 small onion, peeled and diced

1 small stick of celery, diced

1 small red pepper, diced

3 cloves of garlic, peeled and sliced

9 oz lean ground beef

3 tablespoons tomato puree

generous ½ cup cooked Puy lentils

1 bay leaf (optional)

1 sprig of fresh thyme, leaves picked (optional)

¾ cup water or chicken stock

2 handfuls of seasonal greens, finely sliced

FOR THE MASH

7 oz sweet potato, peeled and diced into 1–1½ inch pieces

2–3 large carrots, peeled and sliced

1 tablespoon extra-virgin olive oil

a pinch of salt

PYRAMID: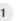

We all need a hearty comfort meal up our sleeves, and this is it for me: creamy sweet potato mash with a rich and tender beef filling, bulked out with lentils for their added fiber, plant protein, and minerals. This is usually a huge hit with little ones too!

Heat the olive oil in a saucepan and sauté the onion, celery, pepper, and garlic for 5 minutes, until soft but not brown. Push the vegetables to one side of the pan, then add the beef and brown for a few minutes, breaking up any lumps with a wooden spoon.

Add the tomato puree, then add the lentils, bay leaf, thyme, and the water or stock. Bring the mixture up to a boil, and then turn down the heat and cover with a lid. Simmer for 15 minutes, then uncover and simmer for another 15 minutes, stirring occasionally, until the sauce has thickened. Taste and season.

Meanwhile, steam your sweet potato and carrots until they are very tender, about 20–25 minutes, depending on the size of the chunks. Drain and mash (or puree with a stick blender), adding a swirl of extra-virgin olive oil and a pinch of salt. Leave in the pan and keep warm.

Just before serving, add the greens to the beef mixture and stir until wilted or cooked.

Swirl half the mash around the bottom of a shallow bowl, then fill the center with half of the beef and lentil mixture.

Place the remaining half of the mixture and the mash into a small ovenproof dish and leave to cool down. Refrigerate overnight. Tomorrow evening, just reheat it in the oven until piping hot before serving with a handful of steamed or blanched green vegetables (use whatever you have left over).

VEGAN ALTERNATIVES

GREEN BEAN, PEA & PISTACHIO SALAD (V)

1 cup green beans

1 cup sugar snap peas

a handful of peas, thawed if frozen

⅓ cup pistachios, unsalted and shelled

4-inch piece of cucumber, seeded and diced

¼ of an avocado, peeled and diced

a handful of baby leaf or herby salad

FOR THE DRESSING

1 tablespoon extra-virgin olive oil

zest and juice of ½ a lemon

½ teaspoon Dijon or whole grain mustard

1 shallot (or ½ a small red onion), peeled and very finely sliced

a pinch of salt and freshly ground black pepper, to taste

PYRAMID:

If they are in season, you could always substitute tender asparagus spears for the green beans here, or perhaps swap some baby broad beans for the peas. Sometimes I substitute my quick pesto (see page 211) for the dressing, which works beautifully well, too.

To make the dressing, whisk together the olive oil, lemon zest and juice, and mustard until combined, then stir through the chopped shallot or onion. Season to taste.

Next, steam or blanch the green beans for 4–5 minutes (depending on their size, they should be just tender but not overcooked). Tip them into a bowl, and then repeat the process with the sugar snap peas and thawed peas, steaming or blanching them together for a further 3 minutes or so. Remove from the heat and add to the bowl. This can all be done ahead of time with the cooked beans and peas left in the fridge until they are needed.

To serve, mix all the salad ingredients together, toss through the dressing, and pile it on to a plate.

LENTIL "COTTAGE" PIE (V)

MAKES: 2 portions

PYRAMID: 4

Lentils have a bit of an unfair reputation for being a rather uninspiring ingredient. Not only are they versatile, wonderfully nutritious, and great value for money, they also combine beautifully with all sorts of different flavors, from fresh herbs (sage, for example) to creamy nut sauces. Or mushrooms and vegetables, as I've done here.

1 tablespoon coconut oil or light olive oil

1 small onion, peeled and diced

1 small stick of celery, diced

1 small red pepper, diced

3 cloves of garlic, peeled and sliced

100g mushrooms, diced

3 tablespoons tomato puree

1½ cups cooked Puy lentils

1 bay leaf (optional)

1 sprig of fresh thyme, leaves picked (optional)

¾ cup vegetable stock

2 handfuls of spinach

FOR THE MASH

7 oz sweet potato, peeled

2–3 large carrots, peeled

1 tablespoon extra-virgin olive oil

a pinch of sea salt

Heat the oil in a saucepan and sauté the onion, celery, pepper, and garlic for 5 minutes, until soft but not brown. Add the mushrooms and fry for a few minutes. Add the tomato puree, stirring it well, then add the lentils, bay leaf, thyme, and stock. Bring the mixture to a boil, and then turn down the heat and cover with a lid. Simmer for 15 minutes, then uncover and simmer for another 15 minutes, stirring occasionally, until the sauce has thickened. Taste and season.

Meanwhile, dice the sweet potato and carrots, then steam until they are very tender, about 20–25 minutes, depending on the size of the chunks. Drain and mash (or puree with a stick blender), adding a swirl of extra-virgin olive oil and a pinch of salt. Leave in the pan and keep warm.

Just before serving, finely slice the spinach and add into the mushroom and lentil mixture and stir until wilted.

Swirl half the mash around the edges of a shallow bowl, then fill the center with half of the lentil mixture.

Place the remaining half of the mixture and the mash into a small, ovenproof dish, and leave to cool down. Refrigerate overnight. Tomorrow evening, just reheat it in the oven until piping hot before serving with a handful of steamed green vegetables (use whatever you have left over).

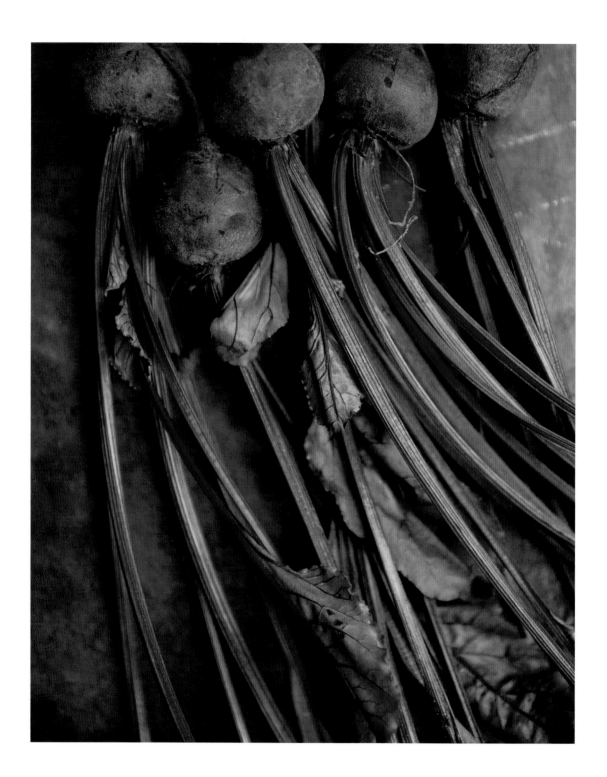

COMPLETE TODAY'S PREPARATION

after supper

1. Take a portion of Beet Hummus out of the freezer (see page 136).

2. Boil two eggs for the Egg Salad on Toast for breakfast tomorrow (see page 291).

3. Prepare your Beet Hummus Salad for lunch tomorrow (see page 292).

for the vegan plan

1. *Take a portion of Beet Hummus out of the freezer (see page 136).*

2. *Soak the quinoa overnight for the Coconut Quinoa Porridge for breakfast tomorrow (see page 294).*

3. *Prepare the ingredients for the Beet Hummus & Avocado Toast for lunch tomorrow (see page 295), although don't assemble it until just before serving.*

Mindful Moment

Sit down at a table every time you eat tomorrow. Eating while standing up can trick our brains into thinking we have eaten less than we actually have. No food should pass your lips unless you are sitting at a table!

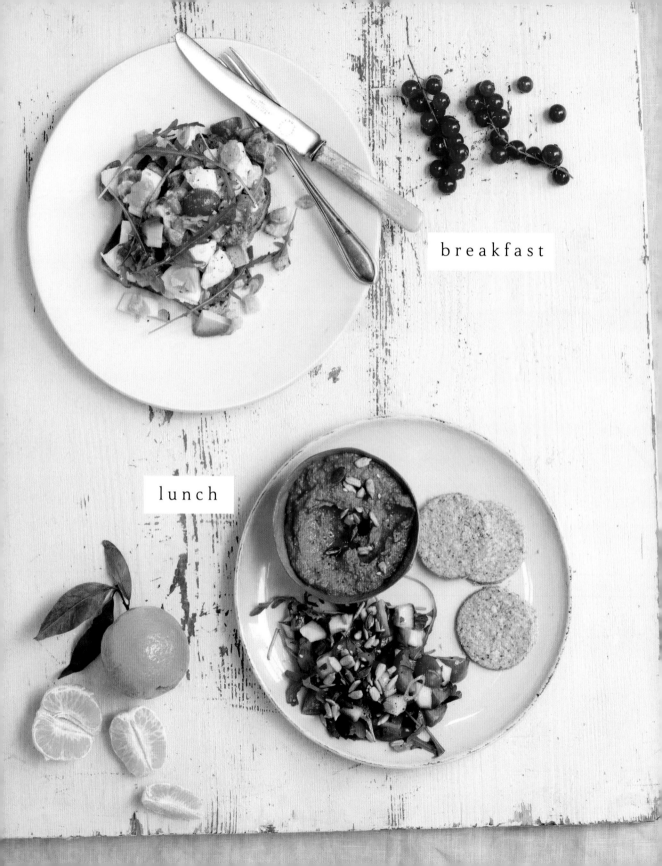

breakfast

lunch

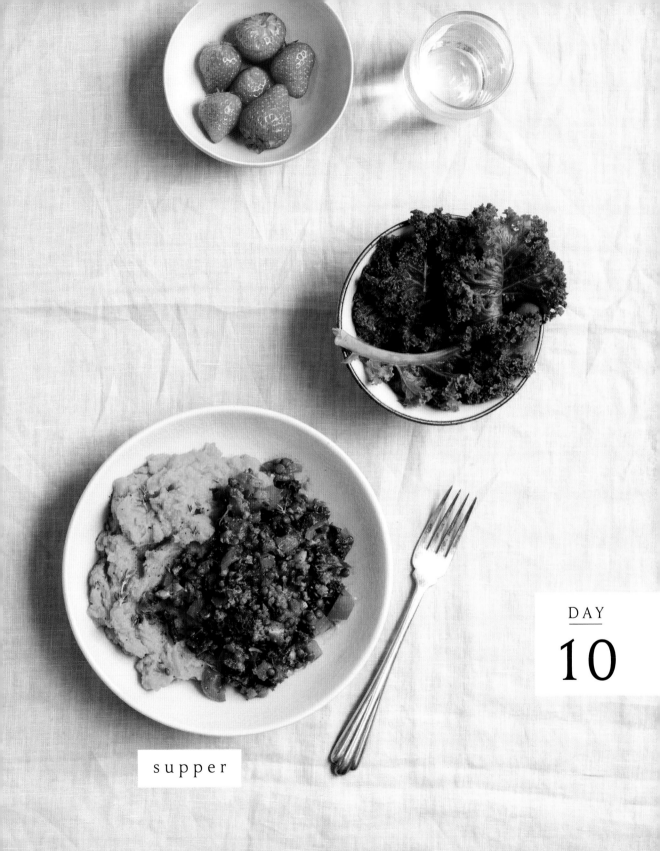

DAY

10

supper

DAY 10

BREAKFAST: EGG SALAD on TOAST
+ 1 PORTION of SEASONAL FRUIT

LUNCH: BEET HUMMUS SALAD (v)
+ 1 PORTION of SEASONAL FRUIT

SUPPER: LEFTOVER COTTAGE PIE with STEAMED GREENS
(see page 281)
+ 1 PORTION of SEASONAL FRUIT

---

vegan alternative:

BREAKFAST: COCONUT QUINOA PORRIDGE

LUNCH: BEET HUMMUS & AVOCADO TOAST
+ 1 PORTION of SEASONAL FRUIT

SUPPER: LEFTOVER LENTIL "COTTAGE" PIE with
STEAMED GREENS (see page 283)
+ 1 PORTION of SEASONAL FRUIT

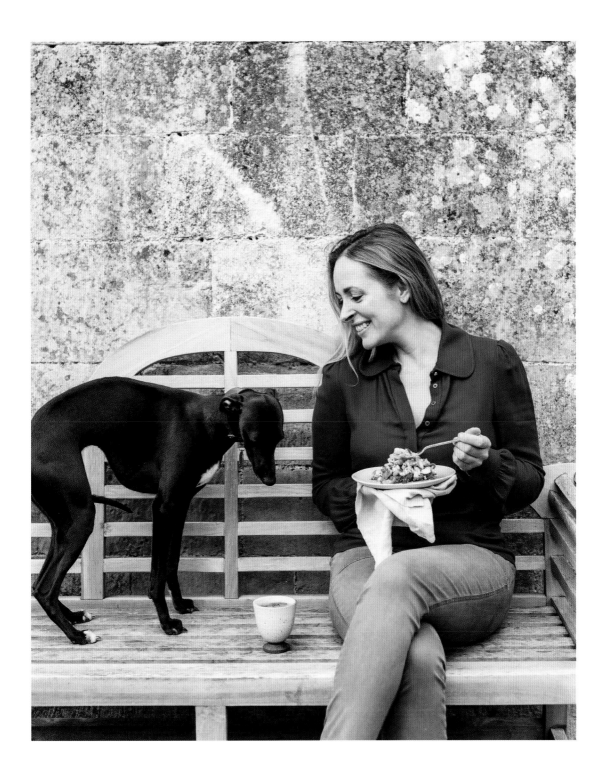

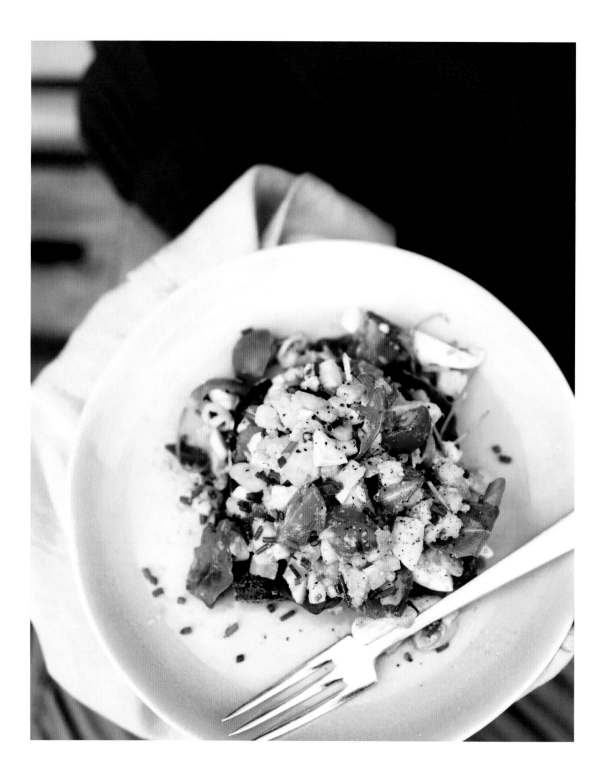

EGG SALAD on TOAST

PYRAMID:

New ways of enjoying classic eggs and toast are always welcome at breakfast—I hope you like this version as much as I do.

2 large eggs

1 scallion, finely sliced

zest of ½ a lemon

a sprinkling of chopped fresh chives

½ a stick of celery, finely chopped

a handful of cherry tomatoes, quartered

¼ of an avocado, peeled and chopped

a handful of arugula

1 tablespoon olive oil

sea salt and freshly ground black pepper

1 slice of gluten-free bread

Boil the eggs for 6 minutes, then rinse under cold water to stop the cooking. Peel the eggs and finely chop them. You could do this the night before if you know you'll be busy in the morning.

Put the eggs into a bowl with the scallions, lemon zest, chives, celery, cherry tomatoes, avocado, and arugula. Add the olive oil and salt and pepper, and mix well.

Toast the slice of bread, and load it up with the salad.

BEET HUMMUS SALAD (V)

a handful of cherry tomatoes, quartered

1 scallion, finely sliced

1 yellow or orange pepper, seeded and finely diced

4-inch piece of cucumber, seeded and finely diced

a handful of arugula leaves, chopped

a drizzle of extra-virgin olive oil

a squeeze of lemon juice

a pinch of sea salt

3 tablespoons Spiced Seed Sprinkle (see page 140)

2 tablespoons fresh parsley, chopped (or basil or cilantro if you prefer)

2–3 gluten-free oatcakes

1 portion of Beet Hummus, defrosted (see page 136)

PYRAMID:

I love the audacious colors of this salad, which (especially once you've made a batch of hummus) is a very quick meal. There are a million and one different combinations that you can try, so feel free to swap or change the suggested vegetables around according to what you have left in the fridge, or what's best at this time of year.

In a bowl, mix together the quartered cherry tomatoes, scallion, pepper, cucumber, and arugula with a drizzle of olive oil, a squeeze of lemon juice, and a pinch of salt. Leave the dressing off if you are making this ahead of time.

Serve the salad mixture topped with a sprinkle of seeds and chopped herbs over the top. Serve with gluten-free oatcakes and a generous dollop of hummus.

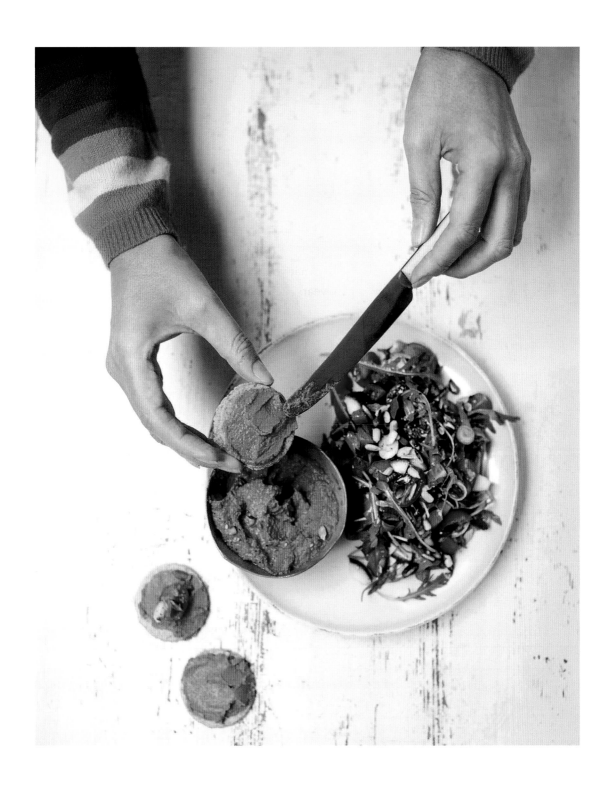

VEGAN ALTERNATIVES

COCONUT QUINOA PORRIDGE (V)

PYRAMID:

This is one of my favorite porridge recipes, using quinoa to replace the oats for a complete-protein boost. Feel free to change the fruit and toppings depending on your tastes and the season. Perhaps try with sliced banana or grated apple instead of the berries, or add a sprinkling of ground seeds, toasted nuts, or some nut butter if you prefer.

scant ¼ cup quinoa

1 cup unsweetened coconut milk (almond or hazelnut milk also work well as alternatives)

½ a vanilla pod (or ½ teaspoon organic vanilla extract)

a pinch of ground cinnamon

½–1 teaspoon sweetener of your choice (honey, maple syrup, or coconut nectar)

1 tablespoon coconut yogurt

1 cup raspberries, blueberries, and strawberries

3 tablespoons chopped nuts or Nut Granola (see page 141)

1 tablespoon grated fresh coconut or coconut flakes, to garnish (optional)

Place the quinoa in a small saucepan with the coconut milk. Scrape in the seeds from the vanilla pod, add the seeds and the pod to the pan, add the cinnamon and sweetener, and stir together. You can do this the night before and leave it in the fridge to soak to speed things up in the morning.

Place over low heat, bring to a boil, then cover with a lid and simmer for 8–10 minutes. Remove the lid and simmer for another 8–12 minutes, stirring occasionally until the porridge is creamy and has the desired consistency, and the grains are tender.

Pour into a serving bowl and top with a dollop of coconut yogurt, a generous handful of berries, a sprinkling of nuts, and the coconut.

TIP: If you are able to get hold of quinoa flakes, available in some health food shops, you can swap ⅓ cup of these in for the regular quinoa. Using the flakes cuts down the cooking time to just 5 minutes, and results in a smoother-textured porridge.

BEET HUMMUS
& AVOCADO TOAST (V)

1–2 slices of
gluten-free bread

1 portion of Beet Hummus,
defrosted
(see page 136)

½ a medium avocado, peeled
and thinly sliced

2–3 tablespoons Spiced Seed
Sprinkle (see page 140)

1–2 handfuls of salad leaves
of your choice

a drizzle of extra-virgin
olive oil

a squeeze of lemon juice

PYRAMID:

This is just the most stunning plate of food—the colors look unbelievable together! Bright, vibrant green avocado against an audacious pink from the hummus is a feast for the eyes as well as the taste buds. Plus, the more colorful your plate, the more variety of vitamins, minerals, and important phytonutrients you are getting in your diet.

You should already have a portion of Beet Hummus in the freezer left over from prep day, so this can be thrown together in no time at all. Once defrosted thoroughly, give it a good stir and it should be as good as new.

———————————

Toast the gluten-free bread well. Spread generously with some hummus, arrange the sliced avocado on top, and finally sprinkle with some toasted seeds.

Serve with a side salad of leaves, dressed with some extra-virgin olive oil and a little lemon.

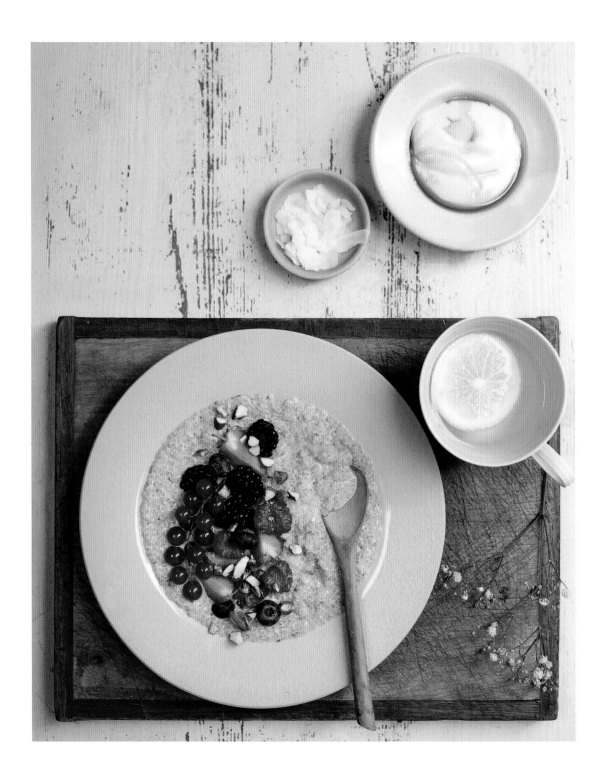

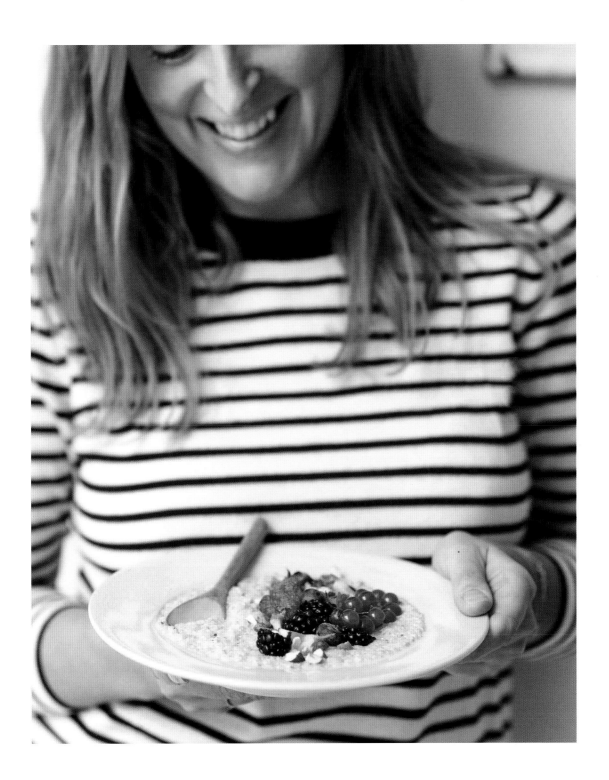

Chapter Five:
NOURISH & GLOW FOR LIFE

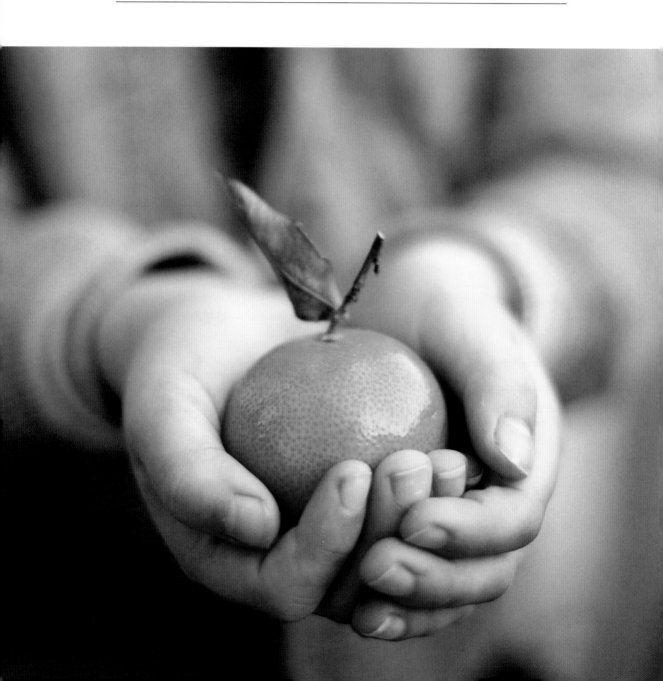

WELL DONE FOR MAKING IT THIS FAR! I hope you are starting to feel a little more empowered and confident about your food choices, and taking to heart the importance of embracing an abundant, varied, and balanced diet.

But how can we keep building on those strong foundations both now and into the future?

I hope this final chapter can help. Tackling some of the common questions—and potential stumbling blocks—we will cement and protect all the positive changes you have already made.

I'M STRUGGLING TO FIND ENOUGH TIME TO EAT WELL. *Any advice?*

This is something I come across all the time. Most of my clients are extremely busy people and struggle to fit eating well into their hectic schedules. But it can be done!

Let me start off with a little tough love here. Time management, particularly when it comes to eating well, is about priorities. If you have time to watch TV or browse the internet, then you have time to eat well. If you really want to improve your nutrition, energy, skin, health, and everything else that comes along with it, then you are going to need to move shopping, food preparation, cooking, and eating right up your priority list.

Of course, there *are* situations in which it can be a logistical challenge to eat well. Given how varied everyone's lives, jobs, hobbies, and other commitments are, it is impossible to give you a personalized answer. I know you have probably heard all the basic things before, not least because many are in this book (using the weekend to prep for the week ahead, taking supper leftovers in for packed lunches, etc.). So instead, try using the following questions to help you find your *own* solutions. They will be better suited to your life than anything I could write!

1. Are you planning ahead?

Planning what you are going to eat over the next few days, even in broad terms, means less time trying to come up with meals, fewer last-minute dashes to the supermarket, and easier preparation.

If you are particularly busy in the mornings, are you preparing your breakfast the night before? Or cooking ahead for the evenings when you know you'll be home from work late?

2. Is your shopping efficient?

Are you shopping every day or just heading out to the store here or there a few times a week? Is it a long round trip to your nearest store? Are you always at work when the stores are open?

- Would a weekly internet delivery of basics be helpful?

- Consider a bulk order of meat from your local farm stand or butcher to put in the freezer—this can be very cost effective, you'll know you always have something to eat, and it is often better quality than what's available in the supermarket.

- Bulk ordering can also be handy for dried goods (the internet is full of great whole-food shops)—things like lentils, nuts, oils, chickpeas, flours, etc.

- Think about joining a community-supported agriculture box program. It means you always have a stash of seasonal veggies to pick from, and most allow you to add on extra items like eggs, fruit, milk, bread, and yogurt too.

3. Have you got the right equipment?

Is your kitchen an efficient place to prepare food? Enough saucepans, a great peeler, decent knives, easily washed cutting boards, plenty of BPA-free storage containers (for all those leftovers and your packed lunches), and a food processor can all greatly cut down on prep time.

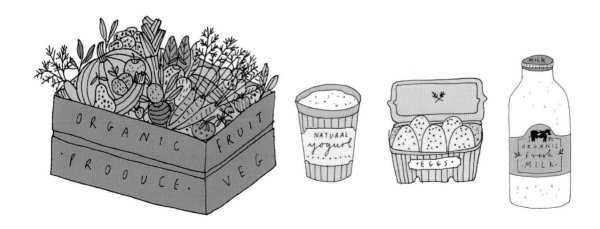

4. Do you prep once, eat twice (or even three times)?

Try to prepare dishes that leave plenty of leftovers for a speedy second, or third, meal. When you are plating up, serve an extra portion into your lunch box—that's tomorrow's lunch done. If you are washing and peeling vegetables, wash and peel some extras too. Freeze leftovers in portions for a homemade ready meal at a later date.

5. Are your recipes overcomplicated?

The Positive Nutrition approach to cooking and eating really can be as simple as piling a load of salad onto a plate, adding some protein (leftover roast chicken, a dollop of hummus, a handful of nuts) and drizzling over some flavor (olive oil, lemon, vinegar, etc.). True fast food! Most of the cooking I do is fast and easy (from fridge to plate in under 5 minutes). So don't worry about trying to be a whiz in the kitchen (unless you enjoy it, of course). No recipe is worth stressing over.

6. Is it really that you are just too exhausted to cook?

You may have enough time in the evening to cook from scratch, but by the time you get home from work (or have put the kids to bed, got back from the gym, etc.), you feel too tired to attempt it.

- Could you make your kitchen a more relaxing and enjoyable space to prepare food in, so that it becomes a less daunting task?

- Are there certain days when you are more tired? Could you plan ahead, so that you know you will have food already prepared on those days?

- Do you have some 5-minute healthy meals up your sleeve (with ingredients in your kitchen) for moments like this? Things like eggs with chopped vegetables (whatever is in the fridge), throw-together salads, or avocado on toast are great. (The "Backup Plan" on page 127 has some simple suggestions.)

I HAVE A BIG PARTY COMING UP.
What should I do?

It is important that we continue to eat a nutritious diet long after we finish the 10-day plan. However, if we constantly restrict ourselves (trying to be "good"), this can go either way: you get to the party and feel unable to touch a thing, which makes you feel both anxious and uncomfortable, or you get to the party and you go "all out" and knock back a little more of everything than you really wanted to. Perhaps in the past you have even skipped social occasions for these very reasons. In all of these cases you can be left feeling worse off than before the party. And that is such a shame, because parties are supposed to be joyful!

When it comes to social occasions and healthy eating, the main thing to remember is that it is not what you do for 1 percent of the time (or indeed 5 percent or 10 percent of the time) that matters. It is what you do the *majority* of the time that is important for your health.

Health is not just physical, but emotional and social too. We need to think a little beyond the pure *nutritional* value of our diets—food can be a very important social bonding tool, as we learned in Chapter One, and a source of great pleasure and happiness too.

So if you have a party coming up, try not to either overly worry about your food or drink choices, nor overly indulge to the point where you feel bad. Embrace and enjoy the occasion. Nourish your social health. Eat and drink mindfully and with grace. Truly enjoy the "worth it" moments without guilt. But above all, try to remember that although food is important, it is not everything. A touch of perspective is never a bad thing.

I HAVE TO EAT OUT REGULARLY FOR WORK.
How can I maintain my diet while in a restaurant?

Sometimes dining occasions are outside of our control, and it would cause offence or jeopardize a business relationship if we refuse to eat "off-plan." There are, however, some simple steps that you can follow that may help you when eating out, particularly during the 10-day plan:

1. Avoid the bread basket.

If possible, tell the waiter that you won't need one.

2. Pass on the wine for now.

Stick to still or sparkling water.

3. Don't be afraid to go off-menu.

It is a running joke in my family that I am incapable of ordering something "as it comes." There is no harm in asking about the possibility of requesting something bespoke.

4. Pick an appetizer instead of a dessert.

Look out for fish, salad, and seafood dishes. If you are eating out during the 10-day plan, avoid dishes containing gluten or dairy for now, too.

5. For your main course, look for a lean protein dish.

Generally this will be chicken, game, or fish. If it comes smothered in cheese or creamy sauce, you can request that this be left off or served on the side.

6. *Add in a pile of vegetables—steamed seasonal vegetables or a green salad or both!*

I usually ask for these instead of potatoes, pasta, or other starchy carbohydrates. Often the restaurant will do this as a straight swap, or you can always order a side.

7. *Politely decline a dessert if you don't really want one.*

Order a mint tea instead—it is amazing how the strong taste of mint can stop you from wanting anything else, and it gives you something to enjoy while your dining companions finish their meal.

These principles can help you to choose the healthiest options, but the odd glass of wine or side order of french fries is just another part of enjoying food.

However, if you are not convinced something is really worth it, even after you've ordered, then leave it (soggy, anemic fries come to mind here!). The same applies once you've had enough. Likewise, if something is utterly delicious, enjoy it and savor every mouthful.

Just because you are eating out doesn't mean you should ignore your body's cues—in fact, these occasions can be the perfect opportunity to practice the "mindful moments" you've learned throughout the plan.

I AM STILL HUNGRY IMMEDIATELY AFTER A MEAL. *What should I do?*

I hope that by reading and working through this book, you have now learned that the only person who can decide on exactly the right diet for you, is you. Tuning into the cues and signals that your body is trying to communicate is therefore really important.

If you are truly hungry after a meal, then your body is telling you it needs more energy. Don't ignore this message for the sake of what is written on a page of a book! Likewise, if you are full and satisfied part way through a meal, then stop eating.

It is, however, important to really check out that this is a true hunger signal, and not something else. Not feeling completely full and actual hunger are very different. With practice, you will become a master at interpreting what your body is trying to tell you, but as with most things worth persevering with, it can take time to perfect.

When I am working with clients who say they still feel hungry immediately after meals, I ask them to go through the following steps before reaching for more food. It doesn't mean you can't have a second portion; it's just a checklist to help you make sure this is *really* what you want.

1. *Have you allowed enough time for the satiety signals to reach your brain?*

   Take at least 20 minutes to see if you are comfortably full before eating more.

2. *Are you thirsty?*

   It is common to misinterpret thirst signals for hunger, so drink a full glass of water and see if that helps while you're waiting for those 20 minutes to be up.

3. *Take a second to "check in" with yourself.*

   Could there be an emotional, stress, or boredom component to your hunger?

4. *What are you hungry for?*

   If you're really just after something sweet, then I do not consider that to be true hunger. It is more of a craving, and in that instance the best thing to do is to walk away and distract yourself until the craving passes (which it will!).

5. *If you are still truly hungry after this, then by all means have some more food.*

   Go for something nutritionally balanced that ideally contains some fat, protein, and carbohydrate—often that simply means a second helping, or check out the snack ideas on page 313–314.

WHAT CAN I DO IF I AM VEGETARIAN OR VEGAN?

It is possible, with thought and planning, to consume plenty of protein, iron, zinc, calcium, and most B vitamins with plant-based eating. The support of a nutritional professional, particularly if you are just making the transition or are a vegan family, is highly recommended to help reduce your risk of deficiencies. The 10-day plan has been created with vegan options every day to try. But here are my suggestions for helping you to eat an optimally nutritious diet as a vegetarian or vegan:

1. Eat as wide a range of foods as you can.

This should help you get a broad mix of vitamins, minerals, and amino acids every day. Try to avoid filling up on foods that are not nutrient-dense (such as processed food and refined grains), so that you have the appetite for plenty of plant proteins and veggies instead.

2. Where are you getting your essential omega-3 fatty acids from?

Omega-3 fats are thought to decrease the risk of heart disease, among other health benefits, and need to be consumed in our diet as our bodies are unable to make them. Certain nuts and seed oils contain the short-chain omega-3 fatty acids, which are beneficial. But the long-chain omega-3 fatty acids (as found in oily fish), do not need conversion by the body. These can also be found in algal extracts. Fish actually get their omega-3 by eating this algae.

3. Eat enough iron!

Non-heme iron (the iron we get from plant sources, dairy, and eggs) is less well absorbed than heme iron (from meat). Furthermore, its absorption can be inhibited by the high amount of phytates (a so-called "anti-nutrient") in a plant-based diet. So, if you are particularly tired, short of breath, dizzy, or pale, it is worth checking whether you have an iron deficiency (your doctor can do this). Many vegans and vegetarians do manage to get enough iron from their diet alone, but (particularly if you are a woman of child-bearing age) sometimes you may need supplementation.

4. Get enough Vitamin D.

Fair-skinned people can make plenty of vitamin D in late spring and summer from just 20 minutes of sun exposure to their forearms and hands each day. Vegetarians will also get some vitamin D from the dairy products in their diet. However, it may be worth considering supplementation with D_3 over the winter months, particularly if you are vegan or have darker skin. Supplements may also be recommended for pregnant and breastfeeding women, children under 5, people over 65, and people who are not exposed to the sun. Speak to a health or nutrition professional for more information on this.

5. If you are vegan, you need to seek out an adequate source of vitamin B_{12}.

We generally only get B_{12} from animal products in our diet. Many products are now fortified (such as plant milks), and yeast extract spread or nutritional yeast flakes contain B_{12} naturally. However, you might also consider taking a high-quality supplement. B_{12} deficiency can potentially be very serious.

6. Include dietary sources of zinc every day.

Phytates can also reduce our ability to absorb zinc, so it's important that you include plenty of zinc-rich foods in your diet. These include tempeh, miso, beans (soak and rinse before cooking to increase zinc absorption), sourdough whole-grain breads, nuts, and seeds.

7. Get enough iodine.

Although we need only small amounts of iodine in our diets, it is still important. Vegetarians may get their iodine from dairy products or eggs. Vegans could use small amounts of iodized salt in their cooking, or include some sea vegetables into their meals (although be careful of eating too much brown seaweed like kelp and kombu—these can be *extremely* high in iodine). Iodine deficiency is particularly concerning for women who are considering pregnancy or who are breastfeeding, and for children. If in doubt, speak to a health or nutrition professional.

8. Build your bones.

Dairy foods are rich in calcium, but you can also find it in green leafy vegetables (except spinach—because the calcium is bound to oxalate, which means that it is very hard to absorb), sesame seeds, or tahini (great for hummus lovers!), nuts, and fortified nut milks.

9. Eat enough protein.

There are all sorts of vegetarian and vegan sources of protein. However, many plant sources do not contain *all* the essential amino acids we need (with a few exceptions, such as quinoa). As long as you are getting plenty of nuts, seeds, legumes, vegetables, and whole grains over the course of each day, however, it's likely you'll be getting everything you need. Eggs are a great source of protein for vegetarians.

10. Seek the advice of a nutritionist or dietitian.

If you are pregnant, breastfeeding, a high-performing athlete, struggling with your weight, or are raising your children as vegetarian or vegan, extra care is needed to make sure that all nutritional needs are met.

Nourish & Glow For Life

NOURISH & GLOW FOR CHILDREN:
the guiding principles

This is not a comprehensive guide to child nutrition (that would be another book!), but here are a few thoughts on cooking and eating with the whole family.

Feeding children is about finding a balance between ensuring they get sufficient energy and essential nutrients to fuel their rapid growth, tolerating their developing independence (or tantrums!), and sharing a love of food. Not an easy task!

Their dietary needs *are* slightly different from our own and will, of course, change over time. Failure to accept new foods and refusal of old favorites is a normal stage of child development, however frustrating it may be. If you are really struggling though, there are nutritional therapists and dietitians specializing in children, including food behavior, who can be a real support.

1. The Positive Nutrition Pyramid and portion guidelines are specifically designed for adults.

Although it is great to aim to get a plentiful variety of whole, nutritious foods into your child's diet, the size and overall balance of portions they need will vary significantly. This is especially true for younger children.

2. No child should be put on a "diet."

Focus should instead be on plentiful fresh, natural foods and limited processed/junk foods, trans fats or sugar. Sugary drinks (including regular undiluted fruit juices) should be minimized—the best drinks for children are milk and water. Healthy fats should not be restricted, particularly if they are coming from sources like organic dairy products, nuts and seeds, olive oil, and avocado, and with all that running around and growing it is important that children get some sort of starchy carbohydrate at every meal (like grains, legumes, or root vegetables).

3. Eat meals together as a family.

Even if this is only achievable on weekends, eating together can encourage children to eat a wider variety of foods, develop important social skills, and help them to learn normal eating behaviors.

4. Try to serve at least one portion of vegetables and one portion of fruit at every meal.

Children should try to get five portions of fruit or vegetables a day—and ideally three of these should be vegetables.

5. Introduce and regularly serve fish (up to 2-3 times a week).

Especially oily fish for essential omega-3 fatty acids. You may find that things like fish pâté (see page 260 for a smoked salmon version), homemade fish fingers (why not try the Fish Goujon recipe on page 242?) or fish cakes go down better than fish fillets.

It is, however, recommended that children (along with pregnant women) do not eat marlin, shark, or swordfish due to the higher mercury content.

6. Keep salt intake very low for the kids.

Try not to add it to your cooking, or leave it on the table. Children do not need much salt. They will get enough from the sodium found naturally in whole foods.

7. Eat breakfast.

Breakfast is vital for their concentration, learning, and memory. Aim for nutrient-dense, low-sugar options. Porridge or overnight oats (see page 196), homemade granola (see page 141), eggs (why not try the Herby Green Omelet on page 259?), or even homemade pancakes are all great options.

8. Have plenty of nutritious snacks up your sleeve for that post-school hunger:

- Plain yogurt with seasonal fruit and honey (they could even make their own "sundaes" with these)
- Fresh fruit and a few nuts
- Hummus and vegetable dippers
- A glass of cold organic milk and a banana
- A matchbox-sized piece of cheese and a couple of oatcakes
- A boiled egg and a slice of rye bread or toast
- Nut butter spread on sourdough toast or apple slices
- Fruit smoothie

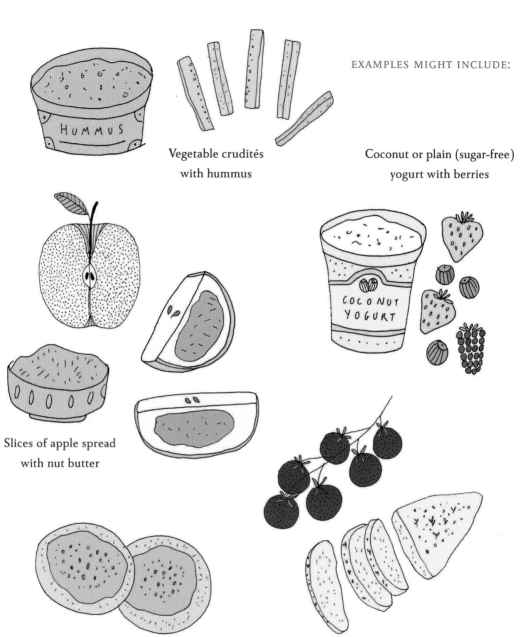

Vegetable crudités
with hummus

Coconut or plain (sugar-free)
yogurt with berries

Slices of apple spread
with nut butter

Avocado mashed with
a little lemon juice on 2 oatcakes
with some seeds sprinkled on top

A few slices of cooked chicken
with some cherry tomatoes

WHAT IF I HAVE HIGHER ENERGY REQUIREMENTS?

If you have higher energy requirements, it is important to get nutrition not just from calories, but from *all* the nutrients that make up a balanced diet. At different phases in our lives, we need different amounts of energy.

One of the most common pitfalls I see in my clients when they have high energy needs is an over-reliance on (often processed) carbohydrates. Although these may have a time and a place (taking carbohydrate gels during endurance events, for example), they can often be rather nutrient-light. I therefore suggest that you try to fulfill your increased nutrient demand by *proportionally* increasing all the food groups. That means more vegetables, fruits, protein, and quality fats, as well as carbohydrates.

You can achieve this using the Positive Nutrition Pyramid and increasing the *size* of your portions to match your requirements and appetite.

If you have very specialist needs (elite athletes or people with medical conditions), I strongly recommend seeing a nutrition professional to help you devise a diet plan which is right for you.

"Exercise is a celebration of what your body can do, not a punishment for what you ate."

A note on exercise

I am not a fitness expert nor a personal trainer, but I do know that diet and exercise go hand in hand, and that regular movement is vital for a healthy mind and body (assuming there is no medical reason why you cannot safely participate). We have explored the diet side of lifestyle in detail, so without going beyond my professional expertise, it seems right to at least consider the importance of exercise too. It is recommended that adults should try to incorporate a combination of aerobic exercise, strength training, and stretching into their week. This is particularly true if you have an otherwise sedentary lifestyle (a desk job, for example).

The benefits of exercise:

REGULAR EXERCISE MAY HELP TO:

- Build healthy bones, muscles, and joints
- Promote mental well-being, and reduce feelings of depression and anxiety
- Prevent falls—this becomes particularly important as we get older
- Boost cognitive function
- Improve our sleep
- Promote and maintain weight loss by burning energy
- Control blood sugar levels in people with diabetes

AND MAY REDUCE THE RISK OF:

- Dying prematurely
- Dying from heart disease
- Having a stroke
- Developing diabetes
- Getting high blood lipids like cholesterol
- Developing high blood pressure (it can also help to lower blood pressure in people who already have high blood pressure)
- Becoming overweight or obese

OTHER BENEFICIAL EFFECTS:

- Building social connections and a sense of community
- Boosting self-esteem
- Learning new skills

WARNING SIGNS:

If you develop any of the following symptoms when you exercise, you should stop immediately and call for help.

- Pain, tightness, or a feeling of pressure in your chest, throat, arms, jaw, or back
- Nausea or vomiting during or after exercise
- Feeling like your heart is fluttering or that you have palpitations, or a sudden burst of a very fast heart rate
- Feeling dizzy, faint, or lightheaded, especially *during* exercise
- Unable to catch your breath

A FINAL WORD

I feel that the quote below really sums up what I have tried to achieve with this book. By walking alongside you as you have explored and experienced for yourself exactly what it means to eat a nutritious diet, I have tried to show you not only how to eat well for a day, a week, or even a month, but how to eat well for the rest of your life. I hope that you now feel able to continue this lifelong venture on your own two feet, gradually building up your confidence and continuing to explore what works best for you.

Perhaps you are starting to feel more energetic, maybe a little lighter, and ideally full of ideas for nourishing meals. I hope that your attitude toward food is gradually becoming more mindful, empowered, and positive, and that you now have the understanding and knowledge to sustain all these changes using the Positive Nutrition Pyramid.

So, huge congratulations for making it this far in your very personal journey. I am sure for some of you this hasn't always been easy, but I am genuinely proud of everyone who has given it a try. Thank you for trusting in my guidance. The rest of your life starts here!

"Give a man a fish and he can eat well for a day. Teach a man to fish and he can eat well for a lifetime."

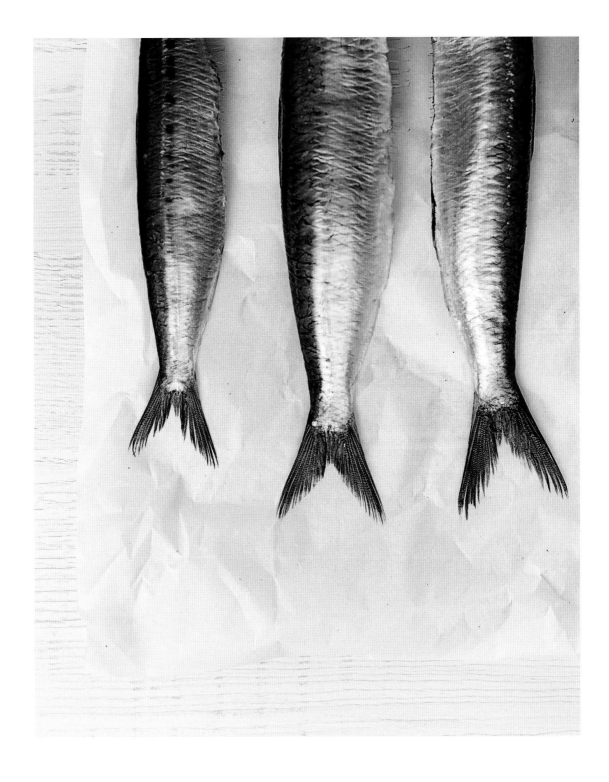

MAIN PLAN SHOPPING LIST

vegetables:

1 eggplant
3 avocados
3 beets (medium) or 2
  packages of cooked
  beets
1 head of broccoli
1 small red cabbage
1 large bag of carrots
1 large bunch of celery
3 red chilis peppers
2 zucchini
1 cucumber
1 endive
2 bulbs of garlic
1 ginger root
4 portions of greens
  (seasonal)
1 bunch of kale
3 leeks
2 lettuce (Bibb)
1 jar of black olives
3 red onions
4 white onions
3 red peppers
2 yellow or orange
  peppers
1 small bag of radishes
  (optional)
1 bag of arugula
2–3 bags salad leaves
  (of your choice)
1 shallot
1 bag of spinach
  (baby leaf)
2 bunches of scallions
1 bag of sugar snap peas
1 large bag of sweet
  potatoes
4 baskets of cherry
  tomatoes (on the vine
  if possible)
1 large package of salad
  tomatoes
Plus a selection of raw
  vegetables for crudités

fruit:

5 apples
2 bananas
1 basket of berries (or
  1 package of frozen
  berries)
8 lemons
4 limes
1 mango
3 oranges
2 pears
Plus 18 portions of
  seasonal fruit (try to
  get a mixture)

fresh herbs:

1 package of basil
1 bay leaf (optional)
1 package of chives
3 small bunches of
  cilantro
1 package of mint
2 small bunches of parsley
1 package of tarragon
1 package of thyme

store cupboard:

1 jar of almond (or
  hazelnut) butter
Apple cider vinegar
Balsamic vinegar
  (optional)
1 can of black beans
Black pepper
1 loaf/package of bread
  (any good, organic,
  gluten-free kind)
1 small jar of capers
2 cans of chickpeas
1 can of coconut milk
  (full fat)
1 jar of mustard (whole-
  grain)
1 package of oatcakes
  (gluten-free)

1 small package of oats
  (gluten-free)
Olive oil (extra-virgin)
Olive oil (light) or
  coconut oil (for
  cooking)
1 package of Puy lentils
  (ready-cooked)
Sea salt
1 small package of
  sultanas
1 small jar of sun-dried
  tomatoes
1 small can of sweet
  corn
Sweetener (honey, maple
  syrup, coconut sugar,
  or similar)
1 jar of tahini
Tamari or coconut
  aminos (best found
  online)
1 tube of tomato puree

nuts & seeds:

1 small package of
  almonds (or hazelnuts)
1 small package of
  cashews
1 small package of chia
  seeds
1 small package of hemp
  seeds
1 package of mixed nuts
1 package of mixed seeds
1 small package of pine
  nuts
1 small package walnuts
1 small bag of flaxseed
  (ground)

dried herbs & spices:

Raw cacao powder
  (or organic cocoa
  powder)
Caraway seeds (optional)

Ground cardamom
Ground chili powder
Ground cinnamon
Ground cilantro
Ground cumin
Garam masala
Dried mixed herbs
Paprika
Pumpkin pie spice
Ground turmeric
Vanilla extract (organic)

for the fridge:

9 oz ground beef
2 chicken breasts
  (preferably organic or
  free-range)
1 carton of unsweetened
  coconut milk (or
  almond milk)
1 large container of
  dairy-free coconut
  milk yogurt (not
  coconut-flavored dairy
  yogurt; could also use
  organic mayonnaise)
12 eggs (preferably free-
  range or organic)
4½ oz jumbo shrimp
2 fillets of white fish
  (e.g., sea bass) (best
  to buy on the day, or
  frozen)
3 lb whole chicken
  (preferably organic
  or free-range)
1 jar or can of tuna
4 salmon fillets
  (preferably wild)

for the freezer:

1 bag of berries (if
  fresh berries are
  not in season)
1 small bag of peas

VEGAN PLAN SHOPPING LIST

vegetables:

1 eggplant
3 beets (medium) or 2 packages of cooked
1 small head of broccoli
1 small red cabbage
1 large bag of carrots
1 large bunch of celery
2–3 red chilis peppers
2 zucchini
1 cucumber
2 bulbs of garlic
1 ginger root
1 small bag green beans
1 bunch kale
1 leek
2 lettuce (Bibb)
1 basket of chestnut mushrooms
2 portobello mushrooms
3 red onions
3 white onions
3 red peppers
2 yellow peppers
1 small bag of radishes (optional)
3 bags of arugula
2–3 bags of salad leaves (of your choice)
2–3 bags spinach (baby leaf)
1 bunch of scallions
1 package of sugar snap peas
1 large bag of sweet potatoes
2–3 baskets of cherry tomatoes (on the vine if possible)
1 large basket of salad tomatoes

fruit:

6 limes
8 lemons
1 mango
2 bananas
5 apples
2 baskets of berries (or 1 package of frozen)
3 oranges
2 pears
Plus 16 portions of seasonal fruit of your choice

fresh herbs:

1 package of basil
1 bay leaf (optional)
3 small bunches of cilantro
1 package of thyme (optional)
1 package of mint
2 small bunches of parsley
1 package sage (optional)
1 package of tarragon (optional)

store cupboard:

1 jar of almond (or hazelnut) butter
Apple cider vinegar
Balsamic vinegar (optional)
2 cans of black beans
Black pepper
1 loaf/package of bread (any good, organic, gluten-free kind)
1 can of lima beans
2 cans of chickpeas
1 can of coconut milk (full fat)
1 jar of mustard (whole-grain)
Nutritional yeast flakes
1 small package of oats (gluten-free)
Olive oil (extra-virgin)
Olive oil (light) or coconut oil (for cooking)
1 package of Puy lentils (ready-cooked)
1 small package quinoa (or quinoa flakes)
Sea salt
1 small package of sultanas
1 small jar of sun-dried tomatoes
1 small can of sweet corn
Sweetener (maple syrup, coconut sugar, or similar)
1 jar of tahini
Tamari or coconut aminos (best found online)
1 tube of tomato puree
1 package organic vegetable stock powder or cubes

nuts & seeds:

1 small package of almonds (or hazelnuts)
1 package of cashews
1 small package of chia seeds
1 small package of coconut flakes (optional)
1 small package of hemp seeds
1 package of mixed nuts
1 package of mixed seeds
1 small package of pine nuts
1 small package of walnuts
1 small bag of flaxseed (ground)

dried herbs & spices:

Raw cacao powder (or organic cocoa powder)
Caraway seeds (optional)
Ground cardamom
Ground chili powder
Ground cinnamon
Ground cilantro
Ground cumin
Garam masala
Dried mixed herbs
Paprika
Pumpkin pie spice
Ground turmeric
Vanilla extract (organic)

for the fridge:

1 carton of unsweetened coconut milk (or almond milk)
1 large container of dairy-free coconut milk yogurt (not coconut-flavored dairy yogurt)
5½ oz tofu
4 oz smoked tofu

for the freezer:

1 bag of berries (if fresh berries are not in season)
1 small bag of peas

REFERENCES

Chapter One: How We Think About What We Eat

1. Robinson, E., Thomas, J., Aveyard, P. and Higgs, S. (2014) "What everyone else is eating: a systematic review and meta-analysis of the effect of informational eating norms on eating behavior," *Journal of the Academy of Nutrition and Dietetics*, 114(3), pp. 414–429.

2. Howland, M., Hunger, J.M. and Mann, T. (2012) "Friends don't let friends eat cookies: Effects of restrictive eating norms on consumption among friends," *Appetite*, 59(2), pp. 505–509.

3. de Castro, J.M. (1994) "Family and friends produce greater social facilitation of food intake than other companions," *Physiology & Behavior*, 56(3), pp. 445–455.

4. Macht, M. (2008) "How emotions affect eating: A five-way model," *Appetite*, 50(1), pp. 1–11.

5. Greeno, C.G. and Wing, R.R. (1994) "Stress-induced eating," *Psychological Bulletin*, 115(3), pp. 444–464.

6. Baucom, D.H. and Aiken, P.A. (1981) "Effect of depressed mood on eating among obese and nonobese dieting and nondieting persons," *Journal of Personality and Social Psychology*, 41(3), pp. 577–585.

7. Blair, E.H., Wing, R.R. and Wald, A. (1991) "The effect of laboratory stressors on glycemic control and gastrointestinal transit time," *Psychosomatic Medicine*, 53(2), pp. 133–143.

Chapter Three: Positive Nutrition

1. NHS Choices (2016) "Healthy Eating," NHS. Available at: www.nhs.uk/livewell/healthy-eating; USDA (2016) Food Composition Database. Available at: https://ndb.nal.usda.gov/ndb/nutrients/index

2. Ros, E. (2010) "Health benefits of nut consumption," Nutrients, 2(7), pp. 652–682.

Chapter Four: The 10-Day Plan to Nourish & Glow

1. Miranda, J., Anton, X., Redondo-Valbuena, C., et al. (2015) "Egg and egg-derived foods: effects on human health and use as functional foods," Nutrients, 7(1), pp. 706–729.

2. Beck, E.J., Tapsell, L.C., Batterham, M.J., et al. (2009) "Increases in peptide Y-Y levels following oat ß-glucan ingestion are dose-dependent in overweight adults," Nutrition Research, 29(10), pp. 705–709.

3. Yang, B. and Kortesniemi, M. (2015) "Clinical evidence on potential health benefits of berries," Current Opinion in Food Science, 2, pp. 36–42.

4. Verbeke, W., Sioen, I., Pieniak, Z., et al. (2005) "Consumer perception versus scientific evidence about health benefits and safety risks from fish consumption," Public Health Nutrition, 8(04).

Chapter Five: Nourish & Glow For Life

1. Sambrook, J. (2015) "Dietary tips for vegetarians and vegans," Patient.co.uk. Available at: http://patient.info/health/dietary-tips-for-vegetarians-and-vegans

2. Burkholder, N., Rajaram, S. and Sabaté, J. (2016) "Vegetarian Diets," BDA. Available at: https://www.bda.uk.com/foodfacts/vegetarianfoodfacts.pdf

3. Duncan, H. (2014) "Healthy Eating For Children," BDA. Available at: https://www.bda.uk.com/foodfacts/healthyeatingchildren.pdf

4. Tidy, C. (2016) "Childhood Nutrition," Patient.co.uk. Available at: http://patient.info/doctor/childhood-nutrition

5. Escott-Stump, S. (2015) "Childhood," Nutrition and Diagnosis Related Care. Philadelphia: Wolters Kluwer, pp. 27–34.

6. NHS Choices (2016) "Physical Activity Guidelines For Adults," NHS. Available at: http://www.nhs.uk/Livewell/fitness/Pages/physical-activity-guidelines-for-adults.aspx

7. Peterson, D. (2016) "The Benefits and Risks of Exercise," Up To Date. Available at: www.uptodate.com

8. Peterson, D. (2015) "Patient Information: Exercise (Beyond the Basics)," Up To Date. Available at: www.uptodate.com

SOURCES

Suppliers

All ingredients in the book are available from most supermarkets and/or health food stores.

Online:
- www.ocado.com
- www.wholefoodsmarket.com
- www.amazon.com

Organic box deliveries:
- CANADA: http://www.uraaw.ca/blog/list-canadian-organic-local-food-delivery-businesses

- UNITED STATES: https://www.localharvest.org

Where I studied:

The Institute for Optimum Nutrition (ION): www.ion.ac.uk

To find a qualified Nutritional Therapist:

For a list of registered practitioners in your area, consult the following websites:

Canada:

- Dietitians of Canada—www.dietitians.ca/Your-Health/Find-A-Dietitian

United States:

- Academy of Nutrition and Dietetics—www.eatright.org/find-an-expert

You could also check out these websites for further information:
- www.functionalmedicine.org
- www.metabolic-balance.co.uk
- www.associationfornutrition.org

Find me at:

www.ameliafreer.com

INSTAGRAM: @ameliafreer

FACEBOOK.COM/AmeliaFreer

EMAIL: info@ameliafreer.com